SIMPLE MORNING YOGA FOR SENIORS

Step by Step Guide to Improve Balance, Stability, Flexibility,loss Weight and boost cardiovascular Health

Leslie K. Lyons

TABLE OF CONTENT

INTRODUCTION

Sandra lives in the peaceful suburbs of a bustling town. Her days were once full of the delights of youth, but as time passed, she became ensnared in a web of age-related discomforts.

Aches invaded her body like unwanted guests, inconsistent weariness clouded her mornings, and the constant aches around her waist, joints, and hips became unshakeable friends.

The absence of regular exercise, along with the weight of life's demands, appeared to put a strain on her aging body.

Sandra wished for a break from the constant grip of agony and tiredness. She wished to reclaim the vibrancy and enthusiasm for life that appeared to have evaded her. In her search for solace, fate led her to a book that would change the course of her mornings, and ultimately her life.

This book contains a wealth of knowledge and advice, as well as a road to freedom from the chains of age-related disorders.

It said Morning Yoga for Seniors, a moderate yet effective ritual for rejuvenating the body, mind, and soul.Sandra began her road to wellness with curiosity sparked and optimism reignited.

She accepted Morning Yoga's teachings with an open heart and eager spirit. With each new day, she began with a sequence of gentle stretches, attentive movements, and relaxing breathwork.

Sandra observed a stunning metamorphosis happen in front of her very eyes as the days grew into weeks and the weeks into months. The pains that had previously plagued her body began to fade, replaced by a fresh sensation of ease and contentment.

The intermittent tiredness that had previously darkened her mornings gave way to a renewed vitality that carried her through the day with elegance and vigor.

The continuous discomfort around her waist, joints, and hips faded into oblivion, leaving only a hazy sense of their previous presence.

Sandra is now a living example of Morning Yoga's transformational impact on elders. She lives to the fullest daily, enjoying every moment with thankfulness and delight.

She has avoided the ravages of age-related diseases by practicing Morning Yoga gently, but she has also discovered a wonderful feeling of vigor and wellness that has no boundaries.

Chapter 1: Benefits of Morning Yoga

Morning yoga has several benefits, particularly for seniors, due to its mild yet effective nature. For seniors, starting the day with a yoga practice may be very beneficial since it promotes physical health, mental clarity, and emotional wellbeing.

First and foremost, morning yoga helps seniors maintain and enhance their flexibility and mobility. As we age, our muscles tighten and our joints stiffen, resulting in a restricted range of motion.

However, the gentle stretches and movements of morning yoga help counteract this by releasing tight muscles and lubricating the joints, therefore increasing flexibility and mobility.

Second, morning yoga enhances balance and stability, which are critical for seniors in avoiding falls and retaining independence. Many yoga postures emphasize balance, requiring practitioners to activate core muscles and focus on stability.

Over time, frequent practice can greatly improve balance and coordination, lowering the incidence of falls and related injuries.

Morning yoga can also help with joint pain and stiffness that many seniors suffer from. Yoga reduces pain and improves joint function by gently stretching and strengthening the muscles around the joints.

Furthermore, the regulated breathing methods used in yoga can promote relaxation and reduce tension, offering relief from chronic pain.

Furthermore, morning yoga promotes mental and emotional well-being in seniors.

The mix of physical exercise, breathwork, and mindfulness promotes calm and inner peace, lowering stress and anxiety levels. This is especially useful for seniors who are going through life transitions or dealing with health issues.

Morning yoga has various advantages to seniors, including increased flexibility, balance, joint health, and general well-being.

Seniors who incorporate a daily morning yoga practice into their regimen can improve their quality of life and retain energy as they age.

Tailoring Yoga Practices for Seniors Needs

Tailoring yoga practices to address the specific requirements of seniors requires careful consideration and modifications to established postures and sequences.

As people age, they may encounter diminished flexibility, balance difficulties, and other health conditions that necessitate changes for a safe and successful practice.

When developing yoga sessions for seniors, it's critical to focus on gentle movements that increase flexibility and mobility while avoiding tension or discomfort.

This frequently entails integrating modifications such as blocks and straps to ensure appropriate alignment and limit the risk of harm.

For example, employing a chair for sitting poses or balancing support might help elderly keep their balance while still benefiting from the exercise.

Furthermore, focusing on breath awareness and mindfulness might improve the whole experience for elders by fostering relaxation and stress reduction.

 Slow, purposeful breathing techniques can help elders connect with their bodies and relax their brains, which is especially useful for controlling anxiety and high blood pressure.

Furthermore, implementing methods that expressly address typical age-related issues might be advantageous.

Gentle backbends and twists, for example, can help relieve spine stiffness, whilst hip-opening postures can enhance mobility and lessen hip and lower back pain.

It's also crucial to offer options and alternatives for positions that may be difficult for elders.

Encourage them to listen to their body and make adjustments as required to create a safe and inclusive atmosphere in which everyone may engage at their own speed and comfort level.

Tailoring yoga practices for elders necessitates a caring and responsive approach that considers their individual needs and limits.

By integrating changes, stressing breath awareness, and addressing common age-related problems, seniors may reap the many benefits of yoga while having a safe and happy practice adapted to their abilities.

Precautions and Safety Measures

When seniors begin their yoga journey, it is critical to prioritize safety and take the required steps to guarantee a happy and injury-free outcome.

As we get older, our bodies may become less flexible and robust, so it's critical to approach yoga practice with care and attention.

First and foremost, seniors should check with their healthcare professional before beginning any new fitness program, including yoga.

This stage is critical for addressing any underlying health issues or physical restrictions that may affect their profession.

Additionally, seniors should tell their yoga instructor of any pre-existing medical issues or recent injuries in order to obtain proper adaptations and assistance.

Props like yoga blocks, belts, and bolsters can give support and stability, particularly for seniors with restricted mobility or flexibility.

These props can assist adapt postures to meet individual requirements while avoiding strain or injury.

Warm-up activities are vital for seniors as they progressively prepare their bodies for yoga practice.

 Gentle exercises like neck rolls, shoulder shrugs, and spine twists can assist enhance blood flow, improve flexibility, and lessen the likelihood of injury throughout the session.

During the practice, elders should maintain appropriate posture and listen to their body. It is critical to avoid pushing beyond their limitations and to acknowledge any discomfort or suffering by adjusting or skipping postures as required. Encourage calm, thoughtful movements to assist elders retain control and avoid overexertion.

Breathing methods are essential for yoga practice, since they promote relaxation and stress alleviation. Seniors should practice deep, regulated breathing to boost oxygen flow, concentrate, and reduce tension.

Cooling down with easy stretches and relaxation poses at the conclusion of the session can assist seniors in easily transitioning out of their practice and promote muscular recovery.

By implementing these precautions and safety measures into their yoga practice, seniors may get the myriad physical and emotional benefits of yoga while reducing their chance of injury and enhancing their overall well-being.

Chapter 2: Essential Morning Yoga Poses for Seniors

Begin your day with a gentle yoga exercise tailored for seniors to improve flexibility, mobility, and general well-being. These fundamental morning postures are ideal for beginning your day with attention and grace.

1. Cat-Cow Stretch: Start on your hands and knees, inhaling as you arch your back (Cow Pose) and exhaling as you circle your spine (Cat Pose). This simple activity warms the spine and improves flexibility.

2. Forward Fold: Begin in a standing posture, hinge at the hips, and gradually drop your upper body towards your legs. Bend your knees as much as necessary to get a comfortable stretch in your hamstrings and lower back.

3. ***Chair Pose:*** Stand with your feet hip-width apart, lift your arms aloft, and lean back as if you were sitting in an imagined chair. Engage your core and thighs while maintaining a straight spine. This position strengthens the legs and enhances balance.

4. ***Warrior II:*** Take one step back while maintaining the front knee bent and aligned over the ankle. Extend your arms parallel to the floor, looking over your front hand, and sink further into the lunge. Warrior II improves leg strength and balance.

5. ***Tree Pose:*** Transfer your weight to one leg and place the sole of your opposite foot on the inner thigh or calf of the standing leg. Find a focus point to aid with balance and raise your hands to a prayer posture at your chest. Tree Pose promotes balance and attention.

6. ***Seated Spinal Twist:*** Sit on the floor with your legs outstretched, then bend one knee and cross it over the other leg. Place your opposite elbow on the outside of the bent knee, then gradually twist your body towards it. This position relaxes the spine and aids digestion.

Incorporating six fundamental morning yoga positions into your practice will help seniors start their day feeling refreshed, motivated, and ready to face whatever comes their way with peace of mind and clarity.

Gentle Stretching Poses

Gentle stretching postures are essential to any senior yoga practice, as they promote flexibility, mobility, and general well-being. These postures emphasize moderate movements that target key muscle groups while combining breath awareness and relaxation techniques.

Mountain position (Tadasana): This basic position helps seniors stand tall with their feet hip-width apart, anchoring the feet and stretching the spine. It promotes posture and balance while instilling stability and relaxation.

Seated Forward Bend (Paschimottanasana): Sitting on a chair or the floor with legs outstretched, elders can slowly fold forward, reaching for their toes or shins.

This stretch lengthens the spine, hamstrings, and calves, increasing flexibility in the back and legs.

Supported Bridge Pose: Using a bolster or folded blanket, seniors can lie on their backs with knees bent and feet hip-width apart.

Lifting the hips softly off the ground and supporting the lower back with the prop stretches the chest, shoulders, and spine while also encouraging relaxation.

Legs-Up-The-Wall (Viparita Karani): Seniors can lie on their backs with their legs stretched against a wall or raised platform.

This position improves circulation, reduces edema in the legs, and generates a state of relaxation and serenity.

Corpse Pose (Savasana): Seniors can finish their practice by resting on their backs, arms by their sides, palms up. This last relaxation posture enables for the integration and absorption of the practice's effects, which promote profound relaxation and stress alleviation.

Balance and Stability Poses

Balance and stability are important parts of yoga practice, especially for seniors, because they improve general physical coordination, lower the chance of falling, and boost confidence in movement.

Incorporating balance and stability poses into a senior's yoga regimen can dramatically improve their health and quality of life.

The tree posture is a foundational posture for improving balance, in which practitioners stand on one leg and place the sole of the other foot on the inner thigh or calf of the standing leg.

This stance not only improves the leg muscles but also needs focus and concentration, resulting in better overall balance. Variations like the Half Lotus Tree

Pose allow for a deeper stretch while retaining stability.

Another useful stance is the Warrior III stance, which entails balancing on one leg while extending the other leg and body parallel to the ground.

This position strengthens the core, improves posture, and increases general stability. Seniors might utilize props such as a chair or a wall for support until they feel confident enough to practice alone.

The Chair Pose, in which practitioners sit back as if in an imagined chair with arms stretched overhead, is beneficial for developing lower body strength and stability. Seniors can progressively increase the time they hold this position to enhance endurance and stability.

Standing Forward Bend Pose, with feet hip-width apart and bending forward at the hips to reach the ground, improves flexibility in the hamstrings and lower back while improving balance. Seniors can utilize props like blocks to adjust their stance according to their flexibility and comfort.

Regular practice of these balance and stability poses not only develops muscles but also enhances proprioception, or the body's knowledge of its location in space, resulting in greater general stability and confidence in movement for seniors.

It is critical to practice these postures consciously, focusing on breath and alignment, and to consult with a trained yoga instructor for suitable advice and modifications based on individual requirements and capabilities.

Relaxation and Breathing Exercises

Incorporating relaxation and breathing techniques into a senior's wellness regimen can significantly improve their overall health.

These techniques not only improve physical health, but they also foster mental clarity and emotional equilibrium.

Seniors can achieve a state of serenity and inner peace by making slow movements and breathing deeply.

Deep breathing is a powerful relaxing method. Take slow, deep breaths, fill the lungs with air, and gently exhale.

Deep breathing techniques can help elders decrease stress, lower blood pressure, and increase oxygen flow throughout their bodies.

Encouraging elders to practice deep breathing on a daily basis will help them improve their lung capacity and respiratory function, which is especially important as we age.

Progressive muscular relaxation is also a beneficial exercise. This entails methodically tensing and then releasing various muscle groups in the body.

Seniors might begin at their toes and work their way up to their heads, observing the sensations of tension and relaxation.

Progressive muscle relaxation teaches elders how to become more aware of and release physiological tension, resulting in more flexibility, less muscular stiffness, and a better sensation of calm.

Guided visualization is another effective approach for helping elders relax and reduce anxiety.

Seniors might use visualization techniques to visualize themselves in quiet, serene places, such as a relaxing beach or a tranquil woodland.

This mental retreat can help elders momentarily disconnect from their anxieties and stresses, generating a sensation of relaxation and revitalization.

Including these relaxation and breathing techniques in a senior's yoga practice can boost the advantages of both.

Yoga is a gentle and accessible technique for elders to engage in physical activity while simultaneously practicing mindfulness and breathing awareness.

Seniors can benefit from a comprehensive approach to health and well-being that includes yoga postures, relaxation methods, and concentrated breathing.

Relaxation and breathing exercises are important parts of a senior's wellness regimen because they promote physical health, mental clarity, and emotional stability.

When combined with a yoga practice, these strategies provide a complete approach to improving general well-being in seniors.

Chapter 3: Designing Your Morning Yoga Routine

Creating a personalized morning routine can dramatically improve seniors' general well-being by adding mild yoga activities that are suited to their requirements.

To improve relaxation and attention, start by creating a tranquil environment, such as with soft lighting and soothing music.

Before beginning yoga positions, seniors can participate in modest warm-up activities to prepare their bodies for movement and avoid injury.

Begin with sitting breathing techniques that encourage awareness and centering. Encourage deep, deliberate breathing, stressing the relationship between breath and activity. This can help seniors relax their muscles and relieve tension, giving them a sense of calm to start their day.

Transition to easy sitting stretches, concentrating on regions prone to stiffness and tightness in seniors, such as the neck, shoulders, and hips.

Gentle neck rolls, shoulder shrugs, and sitting side stretches can help relieve tension and increase mobility, providing a sensation of ease and comfort.

For balance and stability, combine standing postures with the assistance of a chair or wall.

Modified versions of traditional yoga positions such as Mountain Pose, Chair Pose, and Tree Pose can assist seniors gain strength, improving posture, and balance, all of which are important for preserving functional independence and minimizing falls.

Throughout the program, highlight the value of listening to their body and practicing self-compassion.

Encourage seniors to adapt their positions as required, using props such as blankets or blocks for support, and to avoid pushing themselves too far.

The morning ritual with a quick relaxation or meditation activity that helps seniors focus on gratitude and good wishes for the day ahead.

This final minute of calm and thought may leave seniors feeling grounded, energetic, and psychologically ready to face the day ahead.

You may help seniors' physical and mental well-being by creating a morning yoga program that is specially customized to their requirements, concentrating on gentle movements, breathwork, and mindfulness.

Assessing Individual Needs and Goals

Assessing individual requirements and goals in the context of yoga for seniors necessitates a comprehensive approach that takes into consideration age, physical ability, medical issues, and personal preferences.

It is critical to personalize yoga practices to each senior's specific needs while also addressing their general health and safety.

To begin the assessment procedure, the senior's physical health must be thoroughly evaluated. This may include evaluating their flexibility, strength, balance, and range of motion.

Understanding any pre-existing medical issues or injuries is particularly important because some postures or motions may need to be adjusted or avoided entirely.

Understanding the senior's goals and expectations from practicing yoga is critical. Some seniors may want to enhance their flexibility and mobility, while others may want to relieve stress or feel more connected to their community.

Understanding these goals enables instructors to adapt yoga sessions to achieve particular goals while keeping seniors interested and motivated.

It is critical to consider older citizens' cognitive and emotional demands. Yoga can be an effective tool for promoting mental health and relaxation, particularly for seniors who are experiencing stress, anxiety, or depression.

Incorporating mindfulness and relaxation methods into yoga classes can assist elders attain a state of calm and inner peace.

The senior's living environment and lifestyle aspects must also be considered throughout the evaluation procedure.

Understanding their daily routines, physical surroundings, and social support network can provide them vital insights on how to incorporate yoga into their life in a practical and sustainable way.

Overall, analyzing individual requirements and goals in yoga for seniors necessitates a holistic approach that takes into account physical, mental, and behavioral variables.

By adapting yoga practices to meet each senior's specific requirements and aspirations, instructors may help them experience the myriad advantages of yoga while encouraging general health and well-being.

Creating a Balanced Sequence

Creating a balanced sequence for seniors' yoga practice requires careful consideration of their individual requirements and limitations.

It is critical to promote safety, flexibility, and gentle movements while also offering a holistic practice that includes strength, mobility, and relaxation.

To begin, focus on mild warm-up postures to get the body ready for action. This may involve sitting stretches for the neck, shoulders, and spine, as well as mild twists and side stretches to improve mobility and circulation.

Next, integrate standing postures that build strength and stability. Tree Pose, Warrior II, and Chair Pose can help seniors strengthen their legs and core while increasing balance.

To guarantee stability and safety, use objects such as chairs or walls as support.

After standing postures, go on to sitting or reclining positions to continue working on strength, flexibility, and relaxation.

Seated Forward Bend, Cat-Cow Stretch, and Bridge Pose can assist seniors develop flexibility in their spine, hips, and hamstrings while also offering a mild stretch to their chest and shoulders.

Include poses that explicitly address seniors' concerns, such as moderate backbends to counterbalance slouching posture, hip openers to relieve stiffness, and restorative postures like Legs-Up-The-Wall to encourage relaxation and reduce stress.

Encourage elders to breathe deeply and listen to their body throughout the routine. Remind them to adjust their positions as required and to never force oneself into discomfort or pain.

Finish the sequence with a relaxation posture such as Savasana or a guided meditation to allow seniors to fully rest and absorb the benefits of their practice.

Incorporating Mindfulness Practices

Including mindfulness techniques in yoga for seniors can dramatically improve their general well-being.

Mindfulness entails remaining completely present and aware of one's thoughts, feelings, sensations, and environment without judgment.

When paired with yoga, it generates a potent synergy that meets the physical, mental, and emotional demands of older individuals.

For starters, including mindfulness in yoga helps seniors establish a stronger connection between their body and mind.

Seniors can get a better understanding of their body's sensations and motions by focusing on the present moment during yoga postures and breathing exercises. This awareness allows individuals to better understand their physical limitations and avoid injuries, resulting in a safer and more pleasurable practice.

Second, mindfulness in yoga promotes emotional resilience and stress reduction in seniors.

As they focus on their breathing and feelings, they learn to monitor and accept their thoughts and emotions without getting overwhelmed by them.

This non-reactive awareness creates a sense of peace and relaxation, which helps to reduce anxiety and sadness that are frequent in older people.

Mindfulness activities improve cognitive performance and mental clarity in seniors. Seniors who practice mindful breathing and meditation during yoga sessions might increase their concentration, attention, and memory. These techniques also promote neuroplasticity, or the brain's ability to adapt and remodel itself, potentially reducing the cognitive loss associated with aging.

Introducing mindfulness into yoga assists seniors to have a good attitude about life. Seniors can get a sense of strength and self-compassion by practicing appreciation and acceptance for their bodies and skills.

This perspective adjustment increases general psychological well-being and resistance to life's obstacles.

Integrating mindfulness techniques with yoga for seniors provides a comprehensive approach to improving their physical, mental, and emotional well-being.

Mindfulness improves older persons' overall well-being and quality of life by promoting body-mind awareness, emotional resilience, cognitive performance, and a positive perspective.

Chapter 4: Overcoming Challenges in Morning Yoga

Overcoming problems in morning yoga, particularly for seniors, necessitates a deliberate strategy that promotes safety, flexibility, and adaptation.

Morning yoga can be especially good for seniors, as it provides a gentle yet effective way to start the day while also improving general health.

However, some problems may develop that must be handled in order to provide a pleasant and gratifying yoga experience.

Seniors frequently experience stiffness or decreased movement during morning yoga, particularly following a night's rest.

To address this, mild stretching exercises and movements aimed at increasing flexibility can be introduced into the yoga regimen. Begin with easy motions like neck rolls, shoulder shrugs, and mild twists to gradually relax tight muscles and joints.

Another problem is maintaining balance and stability, which can become increasingly difficult as we age.

Incorporating yoga positions that promote balance, such as Tree Pose or Warrior III, can help seniors improve their balance gradually.

Employing props such as chairs or blocks for support may increase stability during standing poses, guaranteeing safety while still receiving the benefits of the practice.

Furthermore, it is critical to tailor the practice to any physical restrictions or health issues. Seniors should listen to their body and adjust their posture as needed to avoid discomfort or harm. For example, utilizing a chair for sitting positions or performing restorative yoga poses with supports can help seniors enjoy the benefits of yoga without placing strain on sensitive regions.

Motivation and consistency might be difficult for seniors, particularly in the morning when energy levels may be low.

Providing a friendly and encouraging environment, whether through group courses or practicing with a companion, can help seniors stay motivated and dedicated to their daily yoga habit.

By tackling these issues with patience, adaptability, and an emphasis on safety, seniors may reap multiple physical, mental, and emotional advantages from morning yoga, improving their overall quality of life.

Dealing with Morning Stiffness

Morning stiffness can become more typical as we age, limiting our ability to begin the day feeling refreshed and agile.

Fortunately, including modest movement routines into our daily routine helps reduce stiffness and increase flexibility.

Yoga has a comprehensive approach to increasing mobility, balance, and general well-being, making it an excellent alternative for seniors seeking to alleviate morning stiffness.

Begin your day with a series of easy stretches and activities that will gradually awaken your body. Slow, deliberate motions should be used to target stiff regions such as the neck, shoulders, spine, and hips.

Begin by gently rotating your neck from side to side, then progress to shoulder rolls and spinal twists to relieve tension and improve mobility.

Next, do a sequence of standing or sitting yoga positions to improve flexibility and strength.

Forward bends such as Uttanasana (standing Forward Bend) and Paschimottanasana (Seated Forward Bend) can extend the spine and stretch the hamstrings, reducing stiffness in the lower back and legs.

Gentle backbends such as Bhujangasana (Cobra Pose) or Setu Bandhasana (Bridge Pose) might help to relieve morning stiffness by counteracting the forward hunching posture and strengthening the back muscles.

Incorporating conscious breathing methods, such as diaphragmatic breathing or ujjayi breath, can boost the benefits of your yoga routine. Deep, regulated breathing relaxes the body and calms the mind, lowering tension and generating a state of comfort.

As you go through your yoga practice, pay attention to your body and respect its limitations.

Avoid pushing yourself into discomfort or agony, and instead look for a mild stretch that feels comfortable for you. Remember that persistence is essential when it comes to receiving the advantages of yoga for morning stiffness.

Incorporating these simple yoga activities into your morning routine may help relieve stiffness, increase mobility, and establish a pleasant tone for the remainder of the day. Begin each day with intention and care, recognizing your body's demands and fostering a sense of well-being that extends beyond the mat.

Addressing Fatigue and Low Energy

Addressing weariness and low energy in seniors with modest physical exercise, such as yoga, can be quite useful.

Individuals commonly suffer a drop in energy levels and exhaustion as they age, which can be caused by a variety of causes such as medical issues, drug side effects, or just the natural aging process.

Engaging in a regular yoga practice designed exclusively for elders can help address these issues and enhance overall health.

Yoga combines gentle movements, breathwork, and mindfulness methods to provide a comprehensive approach to fatigue management.

The practice focuses on improving flexibility, strength, and balance, all of which are necessary for older persons to preserve their mobility and vitality.

Seniors may improve oxygen flow to their muscles and organs by doing mindful breathing techniques, which can boost their vitality and reduce symptoms of tiredness.

Yoga promotes relaxation and stress reduction through meditation and deep relaxation techniques such as yoga Nidra.

Chronic stress may greatly contribute to weariness, thus seniors must learn how to successfully handle stress in order to preserve their energy levels and general health.

One of the primary advantages of yoga for elders is its adaptation to specific demands and physical constraints. To address mobility difficulties or joint stiffness, poses can be adjusted by using props like as chairs, bolsters, or blocks.

This makes yoga more accessible to people of all fitness levels while also ensuring a safe and enjoyable practice for elders.

Yoga not only provides physical advantages, but it also increases mental and emotional well-being, which can boost energy levels.

Gratitude writing or guided visualization can help seniors build a good mentality and boost their sense of energy and motivation.

Yoga is a gentle yet effective way to treat weariness and poor energy in seniors. Seniors who incorporate yoga into their daily practice can enhance their physical strength, flexibility, and balance, as well as their mental and emotional well-being.

With consistent practice, seniors can feel more energy, less weariness, and an overall improvement in quality of life.

Maintaining Motivation and Consistency

Maintaining enthusiasm and consistency in a yoga practice for seniors is critical to receiving the full benefits of this ancient discipline.

Seniors frequently experience unique problems such as decreased mobility, chronic pain, and age-related health conditions, so they must approach their yoga journey with compassion, adaptation, and perseverance.

To stay motivated, seniors might create realistic goals that correspond to their physical abilities and health objectives.

Whether it's improving flexibility, stress management, or general well-being, setting specific and attainable objectives may help seniors stay involved and devoted to their practice

Introducing variation into their yoga regimen by experimenting with new styles, postures, and adjustments can help minimize boredom and maintain interest over time.

Consistency is essential to obtaining the long-term advantages of yoga for elders. Establishing and following to a regular practice regimen can assist seniors gradually gain strength, flexibility, and awareness.

Integrating yoga into everyday routines, whether it's a morning stretch or an evening relaxation session, can help people make it a habit.

To maintain consistency, seniors can use a variety of tools and strategies, including using props and modifications to accommodate their specific needs, seeking advice from experienced instructors who specialize in senior yoga, and practicing mindfulness techniques to stay present and focused during each session.

Furthermore, cultivating a supportive network or joining a yoga group designed exclusively for seniors may give motivation, accountability, and companionship, making the trip more fun and sustainable.

Setting realistic goals, exploring variety, establishing a regular practice schedule, utilizing appropriate tools and modifications, seeking guidance from experienced instructors, practicing mindfulness, and cultivating a supportive community are all part of keeping seniors motivated and consistent in their yoga practice.

Seniors who approach their yoga journey with passion and determination can get the transforming effects of this ancient practice while also improving their general quality of life.

Chapter 5: Integrating Yoga into Daily Life

Integrating yoga into seniors' everyday lives provides a comprehensive approach to sustaining physical, mental, and emotional health.

Gentle yoga poses, breathing exercises, and mindfulness practices can help improve flexibility, balance, and strength while also encouraging relaxation and stress reduction.

Beginning the day with a brief yoga sequence may establish a pleasant tone by waking the body and soothing the mind.

Simple stretches, such as modest neck rolls, shoulder rotations, and sitting spinal twists, can help reduce stiffness and improve circulation. Deep breathing techniques, such as diaphragmatic breathing or alternate nostril breathing, improve oxygenation and can benefit seniors, particularly those with respiratory difficulties.

Taking small yoga breaks throughout the day might help to reduce weariness and improve attention.

Whether it's spending a few minutes performing chair yoga postures like sitting forward bends or ankle rotations or focusing on the breath while doing boring activities, these moments of mindfulness may revitalize the body and mind.

Incorporating yoga into regular activities can also improve functional mobility and help prevent falls. Seniors can practice standing balance postures such as tree pose or warrior pose while waiting in line or doing their daily tasks.

Strengthening poses such as chair squats or leg lifts can be incorporated into ordinary activities such as watching television or cooking.

Restorative yoga positions might help you relax and sleep better at night. Gentle positions such as the reclining bound angle stance or legs-up-the-wall pose can help seniors relax and regulate their nervous systems, preparing them for a good night's sleep.

Overall, seniors who include yoga into their everyday lives benefit from improved physical health, mental clarity, and emotional well-being. Seniors can improve their quality of life by introducing modest yoga activities into their daily routines.

Mindful Morning Rituals

In the peaceful hours of the early morning, elders may go on a restorative journey via thoughtful routines that incorporate the spirit of yoga.

As the sun slowly touches the horizon, ushering in a new day, developing a thoughtful morning practice becomes a holy act of self-care and empowerment.

Start the day by slowly waking your body with gentle, deliberate movements. Enjoy the calm of the morning by engaging in mild stretches and mobility exercises that help the body effortlessly transition from sleep to consciousness.

These motions, which incorporate mindfulness, serve as a gentle reminder to respect the body's own requirements and limitations.

With each breath, elders are urged to bring a feeling of presence and mindfulness into their daily routine.

Emphasizing the significance of conscious breathing, practitioners can soothe the mind and nurture the soul by guiding themselves through pranayama techniques such as deep belly breathing or alternate nostril breathing.

As the body awakens, ask the mind to join the trip with guided meditation or mindfulness exercises.

Simple meditation practices, such as focusing on the breath or repeating affirmations, can help seniors achieve inner calm and clarity.

Seniors can experience a calm flow adapted to their specific needs and skills as they transition easily into yoga postures. Accept the flow of movement as each position unfolds, recognizing the body's inherent rhythms and living in the present now with grace and acceptance.

Finishing the morning ritual with a moment of thankfulness allows seniors to reflect on the joys of a new day and make good wishes for the hours ahead.

Whether via writing, prayer, or solitary contemplation, expressing thankfulness promotes satisfaction and joy, feeding the spirit and setting the tone for a productive day ahead.

In essence, mindful morning routines combine yoga principles with the wisdom of age to promote overall well being in seniors.

Seniors can begin on a voyage of self-discovery by engaging in moderate exercise, aware breathing, and contemplative activities, and viewing each morning as a chance for regeneration and development.

Finding balance throughout the day is critical for seniors' general health and quality of life. Incorporating yoga into their daily practice can help them attain physical, mental, and emotional equilibrium.

Beginning the day with a moderate yoga practice may set the tone for a healthy day ahead. Seniors might start with easy stretches and breathing exercises to wake up their bodies and brains.

This improves circulation, flexibility, and mental clarity, laying a strong foundation for the day. Taking small yoga breaks throughout the day might help seniors stay grounded and balanced in the face of everyday pressures.

These breaks can be as brief as a few minutes and include techniques like chair yoga, which allows them to complete sitting stretches and breathing exercises either at work or on breaks at home. This enables individuals to relieve stress, enhance posture, and recover attention.

As the day develops, seniors might benefit from a lengthier yoga practice in the afternoon or evening to unwind and relax.

This might include a combination of mild yoga positions, deep breathing, and meditation to relax the body and mind.

Practicing mindfulness during yoga sessions can also help seniors become more aware of their bodies and emotions, generating a sense of calm and balance.

Keeping a balanced diet and being hydrated throughout the day enhance the advantages of yoga for elders.

Eating good meals and being hydrated help them maintain their physical health and energy levels, allowing them to participate more completely in their yoga practice and everyday activities.

Overall, establishing balance throughout the day with yoga for seniors entails incorporating short and longer yoga sessions into their routine, as well as attentive eating and drinking habits.

By prioritizing self-care and mindfulness, seniors may improve their physical, mental, and emotional well-being, resulting in a more balanced and happy existence.

Cultivating a Yogic Mindset

Cultivating a yogic mindset in the context of yoga for seniors entails taking a comprehensive approach to wellbeing that includes not just physical postures but also mental and emotional well-being.

Seniors who start a yoga practice might benefit immensely from developing a yogic mentality that values mindfulness, self-awareness, and compassion.

One of the foundational concepts of a yogic mentality is mindfulness, which is being completely present in the moment and aware of one's thoughts, feelings, and body sensations without judgment.

Mindfulness can help seniors cope with stress, anxiety, and sadness, all of which are major issues of aging.

Seniors who practice mindfulness during yoga sessions can improve their attention, balance, and coordination, as well as acquire a deeper feeling of inner peace and satisfaction.

Self-awareness, or understanding one's own ideas, feelings, and behaviors, is another crucial part of developing a yogic mentality.

Seniors who practice yoga can increase their self-awareness by recognizing how their bodies feel during various postures, identifying any areas of tension or discomfort, and learning to alter practices to meet their specific requirements.

Regular practice allows seniors to become more aware of their bodies and have a better grasp of their physical limitations and potential.

Compassion is also a key component of a yogic mentality, urging seniors to approach their yoga practice with love and acceptance for themselves and others.

Seniors may confront particular problems, such as reduced mobility or chronic health concerns, and practicing compassion may help them overcome these obstacles with grace and perseverance.

Seniors who practice self-compassion on the mat can develop a stronger feeling of self-love and acceptance, which can benefit their general well-being.

Cultivating a yogic mentality in yoga for elders entails practicing mindfulness, self-awareness, and compassion.

By adopting these ideas into their yoga practice, seniors may improve their physical, mental, and emotional well-being, resulting in a better and more rewarding existence.

Chapter 6: Yoga for Mind-Body Wellness

Yoga takes a comprehensive approach to mind-body wellbeing, which is especially good for seniors looking to improve their overall health and well-being.

As people age, maintaining flexibility, balance, and mental clarity becomes increasingly important, and yoga offers a gentle yet effective way to accomplish these goals.

Yoga for elders focuses on modifying postures and sequences to meet different degrees of mobility and physical ability.

Gentle stretches and motions can help promote flexibility, improve joint health, and relieve the stiffness that comes with age. Using yoga supports like blocks, belts, and chairs improves accessibility and safety while practicing.

Beyond the physical advantages, yoga helps mental health by fostering mindfulness and stress reduction.

Breathing exercises, or pranayama, promote relaxation, tranquility, and mental clarity, allowing elders to cope with daily challenges and create a stronger feeling of inner peace.

Including meditation techniques in yoga sessions improves attention, concentration, and emotional resilience, promoting a positive attitude on life.

Yoga provides a social outlet for seniors, encouraging a sense of belonging and connection with others. Group yoga courses provide chances for social engagement, support, and camaraderie, which can help battle feelings of loneliness and isolation that are common in older adults.

Incorporating yoga into a senior's regimen increases energy and improves quality of life. Regular practice improves posture, balance, and coordination, which reduces the likelihood of falls and accidents.

Yoga's gentle nature also makes it a safe and effective form of exercise for seniors suffering from chronic diseases like arthritis or osteoporosis.

Yoga offers a holistic approach to mind-body wellbeing for seniors, with physical, mental, and social advantages.

Seniors who incorporate yoga into their daily routine can improve their overall health, energy, and quality of life, allowing them to age gracefully while also living a happy and active existence.

Understanding the Mind-Body Connection

Seniors who practice yoga must understand the delicate interaction between mind and body. Yoga includes a variety of physical postures, breathing exercises, and meditation practices that work together to enhance total well-being.

Seniors can benefit from the mind-body link in a variety of ways, including improved physical health, mental clarity, and emotional stability.

Yoga's physical poses, or asanas, assist seniors improve their flexibility, strength and balance. These postures activate several muscle groups and increase blood circulation, which is essential for preserving joint health and mobility as one ages.

Regular yoga practice can help seniors minimize stiffness and discomfort, and improve their overall physical performance.

Breathing techniques, such as pranayama, are essential components of yoga practice that promote relaxation and stress reduction.

Deep, deliberate breathing practices can help elders relax their nervous systems, reduce anxiety, and increase lung capacity.

Seniors who include mindful breathing into their daily practice can improve their respiratory health while also cultivating a sense of inner calm and tranquility.

Meditation practices in yoga help seniors develop present-moment mindfulness and mental clarity.

Meditation activities, such as mindfulness meditation or guided visualization, can assist seniors quiet their minds, decrease stress, and improve cognitive performance. Seniors might improve their emotional resilience and brain sharpness by practicing meditation on a regular basis.

The mind-body connection in yoga extends beyond physical exercises and breath practice; it entails developing a deeper awareness of oneself and adopting a holistic approach to health and wellness.

Seniors who practice yoga not only enhance their physical health, but they also acquire more self-awareness and emotional fortitude.

Yoga for elders is a holistic approach to improving health and well-being by fostering the mind-body connection.

Seniors can enhance their physical health, mental clarity, and emotional stability by practicing physical postures, breathing exercises, and meditation techniques, thereby increasing their overall quality of life.

Exposed secret to achieve faster body Health for seniors

A specialized strategy is required to achieve quicker bodily health for elders, prioritizing safety, sustainability, and addressing unique age-related factors. **Here's a thorough breakdown:**

Consultation and Assessment: Before starting any new health or fitness plan, elders should speak with their doctor for a thorough evaluation.

This evaluation should take into account the current health state, medical history, pre-existing illnesses (e.g., arthritis, osteoporosis), medicines, and any limitations or concerns.

tailored activity Plan: Using the exam, seniors can collaborate with a fitness consultant or physical therapist to create a tailored activity plan. This program should

include a variety of cardiovascular activities (e.g., walking, swimming), strength training (e.g., resistance bands, bodyweight exercises), flexibility exercises (e.g., yoga, tai chi), and balancing exercises.
The plan should be adapted to each individual's talents, goals, and any pre-existing health concerns or limits.

Gradual Progress: Seniors should begin cautiously and progressively increase the intensity, duration, and frequency of their exercise sessions over time

This slow approach helps to prevent injuries while also allowing the body to adapt and improve over time.

Focus on Functional Movements: Include exercises that increase functional movements used in everyday tasks such as squatting, bending, reaching, lifting, and walking.

Functional training increases mobility, flexibility, and general functional ability, making daily chores easier and lowering the risk of falls and accidents.

Proper Nutrition: Seniors should eat a well-balanced diet rich in nutrients to maintain their overall health and energy levels.

This contains an abundance of fruits, vegetables, whole grains, lean meats, and healthy fats. Adequate hydration is also required for peak health and performance.

Rest and Recovery: Seniors should emphasize appropriate rest and recovery time in between exercise sessions to allow their bodies to repair and regenerate.

This includes getting adequate sleep each night and scheduling rest days into their fitness schedule as needed.

Social Support and Engagement: Maintaining social ties and being involved with friends, family, and community groups can benefit seniors' overall health and wellness.

Social support gives inspiration, encouragement, and a sense of belonging, which can help you stick to a healthy lifestyle.

Regular Monitoring and Adjustments: Seniors should track their progress, listen to their body, and make changes to their exercise plan as needed.

This might include altering activities, reducing intensity levels, or getting advice from a fitness expert or healthcare specialist.

Seniors may attain and maintain better physical health in a safe and sustainable way by adhering to these principles and adopting them into their everyday lives.

Remember, it's never too late to start prioritizing your health and wellness!

Cultivating Emotional Resilience

Cultivating emotional resilience with yoga for seniors entails a thoughtful combination of movement, breath, and mindfulness to promote inner strength and flexibility in the face of life's adversities.

As people age, they may face a variety of physical restrictions and mental challenges, making it critical to learn techniques for managing these changes with grace and fortitude.

Yoga takes a comprehensive approach to emotional well-being, including moderate physical postures, breathwork, meditation, and relaxation techniques.

Seniors can improve their emotional resilience through frequent practice, building a greater sense of self-awareness, self-compassion, and acceptance of their bodies and limits.

One important part of yoga for elders is the emphasis on mindfulness. Seniors might acquire a more balanced and sympathetic view of themselves and others by practicing present-moment awareness during yoga sessions.

This mindfulness exercise can be especially useful for dealing with stress, worry, and feelings of loneliness or isolation that are typical in old age.

Another significant aspect of yoga for elders is the emphasis on gentle movement and breathing exercises. Seniors are urged to walk slowly and thoughtfully through a sequence of postures, with an emphasis on breath awareness to relieve tension and promote relaxation.

This moderate approach to movement not only increases flexibility, strength, and balance, but it also helps seniors gain confidence in their bodies and adaptability to change.

Yoga for elders frequently includes techniques like guided meditation and deep relaxation to enhance emotional well-being.

These activities provide seniors with a secure environment to reconnect with their inner selves, cultivate appreciation, and discover moments of peace and calm despite life's difficulties.

Yoga for elders is a comprehensive approach to emotional resilience, including mindfulness, moderate movement, breathwork, and relaxation methods.

Regular practice can help seniors improve their capacity to face life's obstacles with grace, acceptance, and inner strength.

Enhancing Cognitive Function

Yoga for elders improves cognitive function by using a comprehensive approach that considers both physical and mental well-being.

Cognitive decline can occur as people age for a variety of reasons, including less brain plasticity and increased stress. However, practicing yoga can help with cognitive performance and general brain health.

Yoga combines physical postures (asanas), breathing methods (pranayama), and meditation, all of which can improve cognitive performance.

Asanas increase flexibility, strength, and balance, all of which are necessary for seniors to retain mobility and lower their risk of falling.

Certain yoga postures, such as Downward-Facing Dog and Warrior II, demand focus and concentration, which might assist improve cognitive abilities.

Pranayama, or regulated breathing techniques, are another important component of yoga that might improve cognitive performance.

Deep breathing techniques such as diaphragmatic breathing and alternate nostril breathing assist to relax the mind, reduce stress, and enhance oxygenation to the brain.

These routines have been demonstrated to improve attention, memory, and cognitive ability. Meditation, which is frequently included into yoga practice, is an effective method for boosting cognitive function in seniors.

Meditation approaches such as mindfulness and loving-kindness meditation help improve attention, working memory, and emotional control.

Regular meditation practice has also been related to anatomical changes in the brain, such as increased gray matter density in memory and executive functions.

In addition to the physical and emotional advantages of yoga, practicing in a group environment can improve seniors' cognitive well-being.

Participating in yoga courses encourages social connection, which is necessary for cognitive stimulation and emotional support.

Yoga combines physical movement, breathwork, meditation, and social involvement to provide a complete approach to improving cognitive function in seniors. Seniors who incorporate yoga into their practice can improve their cognitive ability, brain health, and quality of life.

Chapter 7: Sustaining Your Morning Yoga Practice

Beginning your day with soft movements and attentive breathing might help to create a pleasant tone for the remainder of the day.

Including yoga in seniors' daily routines provides several physical and emotional health advantages.

However, maintaining this practice needs commitment and a few modifications to assure safety and comfort.

To maintain your morning yoga practice as a senior, consider consistency above pushing yourself too hard. Begin by providing a friendly practicing environment that is devoid of distractions and risks.

A peaceful location with a non-slip mat and supporting props can help you stay stable and comfortable while doing postures.

To build a sense of serenity and presence during your practice, focus on seamless transitions and focused breathing.

Focus on soft motions that build flexibility, balance, and strength without strain. Investigate adaptations and changes in positions to meet any physical restrictions or pain.

Consistency is essential to receiving the advantages of yoga for elders. Set reasonable goals and commit to a consistent practice regimen that corresponds to your energy level and daily routine.

Whether it's a quick workout every morning or longer sessions a few times a week, find a rhythm that works for you and stick to it.

Seek help from skilled teachers who have expertise teaching yoga to elders. They can provide unique changes and direction to guarantee a safe and successful practice based on your specific requirements and skills.

Throughout your practice, remember to listen to and heed your body's messages. If a stance is difficult or painful, simply back off or consider alternate possibilities.

 Be patient with yourself and recognize your accomplishments, no matter how tiny.

Incorporating mindfulness and appreciation into your daily yoga routine might increase the advantages for seniors. Develop a sense of self-compassion and gratitude for your body's knowledge and perseverance.

Seniors can improve their general well-being and vigor for the day by cultivating a consistent morning yoga program that includes mindfulness and self-care.

Adjusting Yoga Practices with Age

Individuals' bodies change as they age, affecting their capacity to participate in particular physical activities, such as yoga.

It is critical to alter yoga techniques to meet these changes and ensure that seniors continue to get the benefits of this ancient practice.

For starters, arthritis or joint stiffness can cause elderly to lose flexibility and movement. As a result, yoga poses should be changed to be less strenuous on the joints and gradually increase flexibility.

For example, employing props such as yoga blocks or straps can help you achieve postures without hurting your muscles or joints.

Second, as we age, balance becomes more vital for avoiding falls and maintaining stability. Balance-focused postures, such as Tree Pose and Warrior III, can assist seniors improve their balance and coordination.

Furthermore, performing sitting yoga postures or utilizing a chair for support helps improve stability while still receiving the benefits of yoga.

Third, breathing exercises, also known as pranayama, are essential for elderly yoga practitioners. Deep breathing exercises can help you decrease stress, enhance lung function, and relax.

Simple methods such as diaphragmatic breathing or alternate nostril breathing can simply be included into a senior's yoga practice.

Furthermore, mindfulness and meditation techniques help seniors improve their mental clarity, attention, and emotional well-being.

Mindfulness practices like body scans and guided imagery can help seniors connect with their bodies and manage any discomfort or suffering they may feel while doing yoga.

Elders should listen to their bodies and exercise self-care throughout yoga sessions. Encourage adaptations or breaks as required and practice yoga at a comfortable pace, to assist seniors realize the physical, mental, and emotional benefits of yoga while respecting their bodies' limits.

Modifying postures, concentrating on balance and stability, including breathing exercises and mindfulness methods, and engaging in self-care are all part of adapting yoga practices for elders.

By adapting yoga sessions to seniors' requirements, they may continue to reap the numerous benefits of this ancient practice far into their golden years.

Embracing Yoga as a Lifestyle

Embracing a yogic lifestyle has significant benefits for seniors, providing a comprehensive approach to physical, mental, and emotional health.

For elders, yoga is a gentle yet effective way to preserve flexibility, improve balance, and increase general mobility. Yoga promotes body-mind balance by incorporating conscious movement and breath awareness, resulting in increased vigor and resilience.

Adaptability is an important feature of yoga for elders. Poses may be modified and props added to meet different degrees of mobility and physical ability.

This inclusion enables seniors to safely practice yoga, regardless of their present fitness level or health status.

Yoga's mild nature makes it suitable for seniors with joint problems, arthritis, or other age-related concerns.

Beyond the physical advantages, yoga promotes mental and emotional well-being. The practice of mindfulness in yoga allows seniors to create present-moment awareness, which reduces tension and anxiety.

Breathing exercises, or pranayama, encourage relaxation and peace, whereas meditation promotes mental clarity and emotional resilience. These techniques enable elders to face life's obstacles with more calm and grace.

Yoga also promotes a sense of community and belonging, particularly in specialist courses for elders. Sharing practice with peers fosters a friendly atmosphere in which people may interact, mingle, and discuss their experiences.

This sense of community improves the general well-being of elders by minimizing feelings of isolation and loneliness.

Incorporating yoga into daily life extends beyond the limitations of the yoga mat. It entails embracing yogic ideals like compassion, appreciation, and self-awareness. Seniors who practice yoga as a lifestyle become more aware of their bodies, thoughts, and the environment around them.

This increased awareness improves their life, giving them a greater feeling of fulfillment and purpose throughout their golden years.

Embracing yoga as a lifestyle provides seniors with a road to overall well-being. Yoga improves physical health, mental clarity, emotional resilience, and social relationships by using flexible practices and mindful concepts.

By incorporating yoga into their everyday lives, seniors may create vigor, pleasure, and a profound feeling of fulfillment as they age gracefully.

Building Community and Support

Developing a supportive community around yoga for seniors is critical to creating a secure, inclusive, and powerful atmosphere in which participants may develop physically, psychologically, and emotionally.

This supportive network not only improves the overall yoga experience, but it also plays an important role in encouraging social connectivity and emotional well-being among seniors.

Offering specific lessons targeted to their individual needs and skills is one way to foster community and support within a yoga for seniors program.

These programs might focus on gentle movements, stretching, and breathing exercises that address the unique physical limits and health issues that older people face. Seniors are more likely to engage actively and make meaningful connections with their peers if they are in an environment where they feel comfortable and secure in their work.

In addition to specialized sessions, including social components in the yoga program can help to create community relationships.

This might involve arranging frequent group trips, workshops, or social meetings where members can share their yoga-related experiences, recommendations, and observations.

Building a sense of camaraderie and companionship among seniors not only improves their yoga practice, but also adds to their general sense of belonging and security.

Furthermore, building a supporting network of skilled teachers and personnel that understand the special requirements of elders is critical. These teachers should be skilled at adjusting yoga postures and sequences to the diverse physical abilities and health issues that older individuals typically face.

Seniors can feel empowered to explore their practice safely and confidently when a supportive and inclusive teaching atmosphere is created, knowing that they are receiving specific attention and direction.

Developing community and support in a yoga for elders program extends beyond the physical practice on the mat. It entails providing a friendly and inclusive environment in which elders feel respected, encouraged, and motivated to continue their path to holistic well-being.

Yoga may be a transforming and uplifting experience for seniors by fostering meaningful connections, providing customized training, and encouraging social participation.

CONCLUSION

Yoga for elders has emerged as a diverse and extremely effective practice that promotes physical, mental, and emotional well-being in this group.

Yoga, which combines gentle exercises, breathwork, and mindfulness methods, provides seniors with a comprehensive approach to preserving and enhancing their overall health.

Physically, yoga promotes flexibility, balance, and strength, all of which are essential components of good aging.

Regular yoga practice can help seniors offset the effects of aging on the musculoskeletal system, lower the risk of falls, and improve mobility, boosting independence and quality of life.

The emphasis on precise alignment and regulated movements reduces the chance of injury, making yoga a safe and accessible form of exercise for older individuals of various physical abilities.

Yoga is an effective stress-reduction and relaxation technique. The combination of breath awareness and meditation practices promotes a sense of peace and tranquility, assisting seniors in managing the daily tensions and problems associated with aging.

This component of yoga is especially important given the high frequency of stress-related illnesses among older people, such as anxiety, depression, and cognitive impairment. Seniors who incorporate yoga into their regimen can improve their mental resilience and emotional well-being, resulting in a more positive attitude on life.

Furthermore, yoga fosters a feeling of community and belonging as seniors gather in a supportive setting to practice and interact with one another. This social side of yoga is crucial, especially for seniors who may be feeling social isolation or loneliness.

Seniors who participate in group seminars or workshops not only benefit from the supervision of experienced teachers, but they also build important relationships with their peers, fostering a feeling of community and mutual support.

Yoga for elders is a complete approach to healthy aging that addresses the physical, mental, and social aspects of well-being.

Seniors who incorporate yoga into their daily routine can improve their overall quality of life, preserve their independence, and build a feeling of vigor and resilience as they age.

As research continues to unearth the numerous advantages of yoga for older persons, including it into senior wellness programs and community efforts offers enormous potential for promoting healthy aging and improving the lives of seniors throughout the world.

THANK YOU PAGE

Thank you for selecting this book. Your support is really appreciated. Similarly, I am grateful for the purchase of this book.

Your input is valuable; please share your ideas in a review. It serves as a reference for future improvements. Enjoy reading and utilizing it!

Workout plan to help you track and achieve your desired result

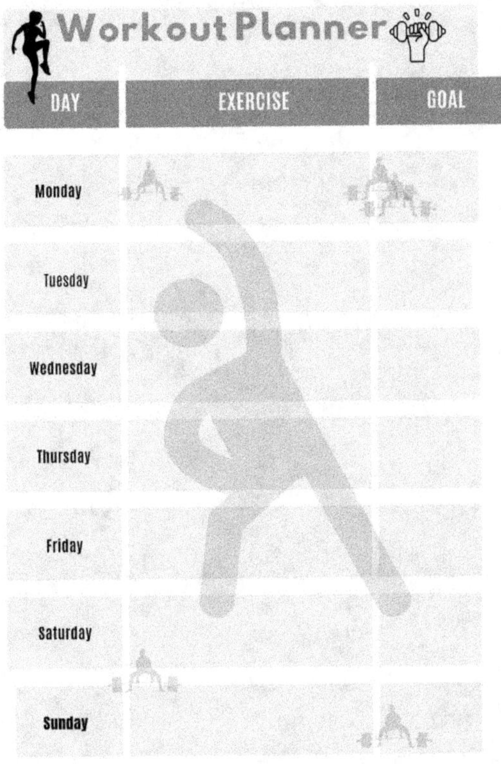

Workout Planner

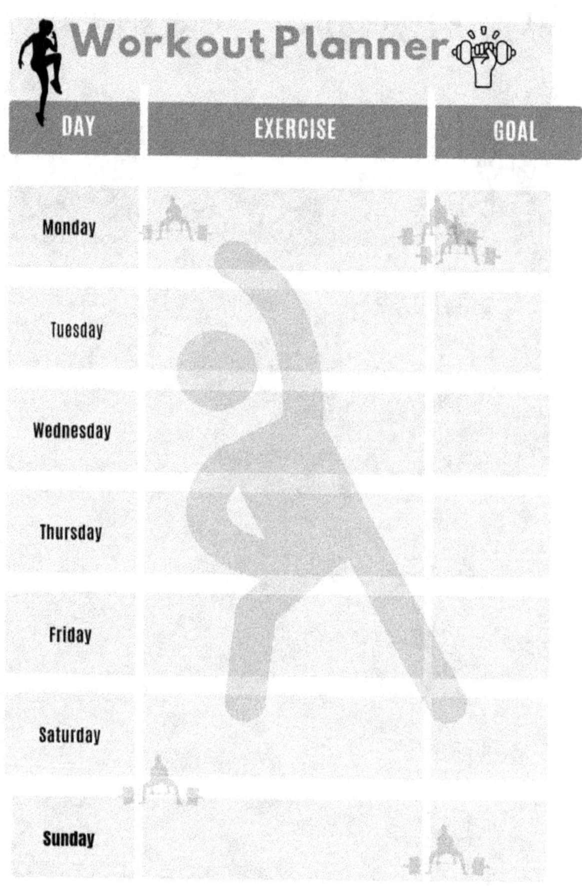

DAY	EXERCISE	GOAL
Monday		
Tuesday		
Wednesday		
Thursday		
Friday		
Saturday		
Sunday		

Workout Planner

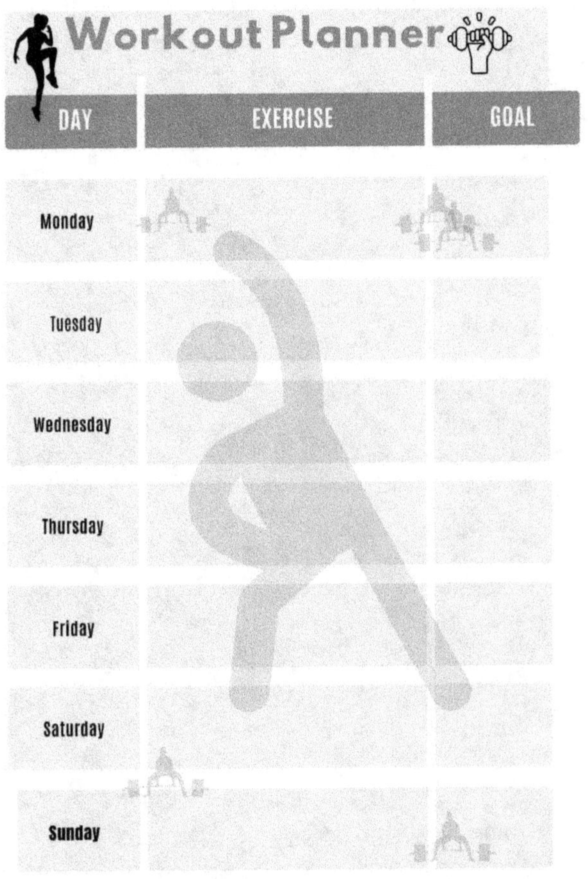

DAY	EXERCISE	GOAL
Monday		
Tuesday		
Wednesday		
Thursday		
Friday		
Saturday		
Sunday		

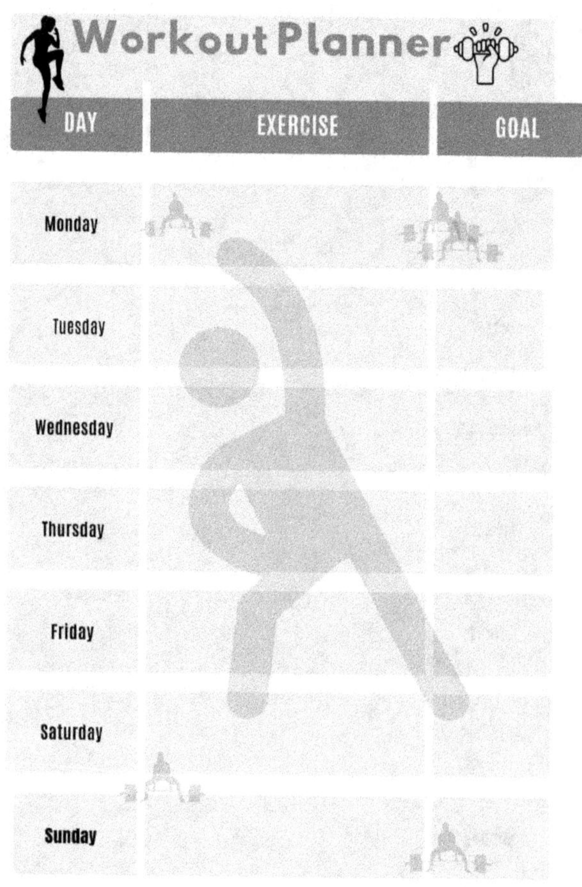

Workout Planner
DAY
EXERCISE
GOAL
Monday
Tuesday
Wednesday
Thursday
Friday
Saturday
Sunday

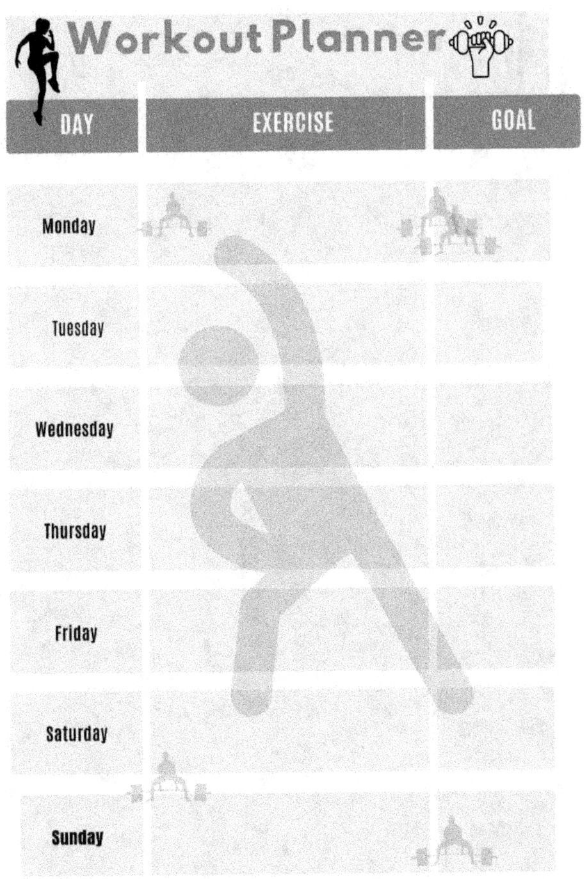
Workout Planner
DAY
EXERCISE
GOAL
Monday
Tuesday
Wednesday
Thursday
Friday
Saturday
Sunday

Workout Planner

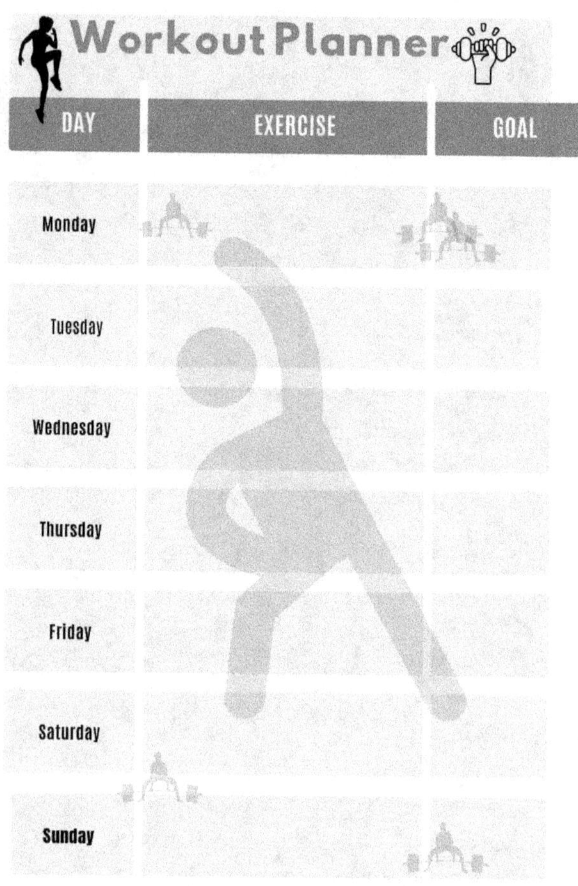

DAY	EXERCISE	GOAL
Monday		
Tuesday		
Wednesday		
Thursday		
Friday		
Saturday		
Sunday		

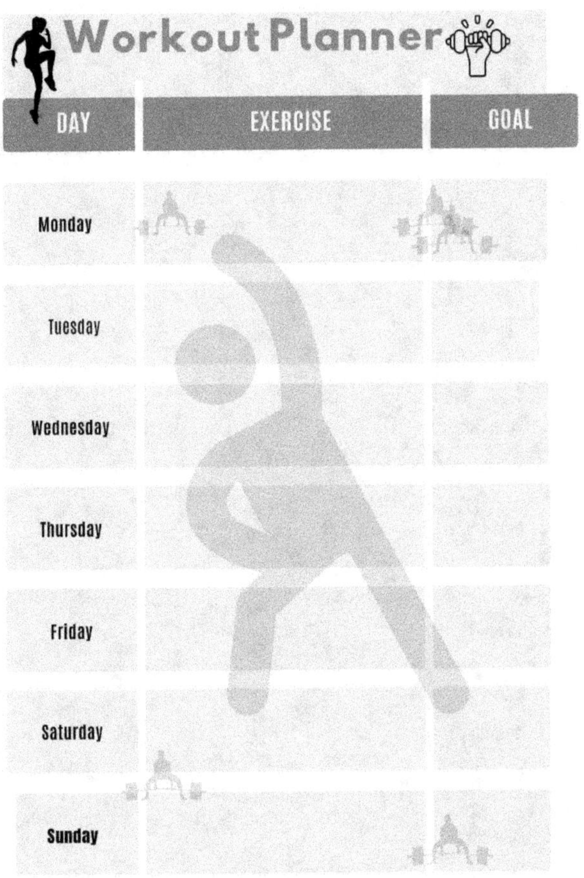

Workout Planner
DAY
EXERCISE
GOAL
Monday
Tuesday
Wednesday
Thursday
Friday
Saturday
Sunday

Workout Planner

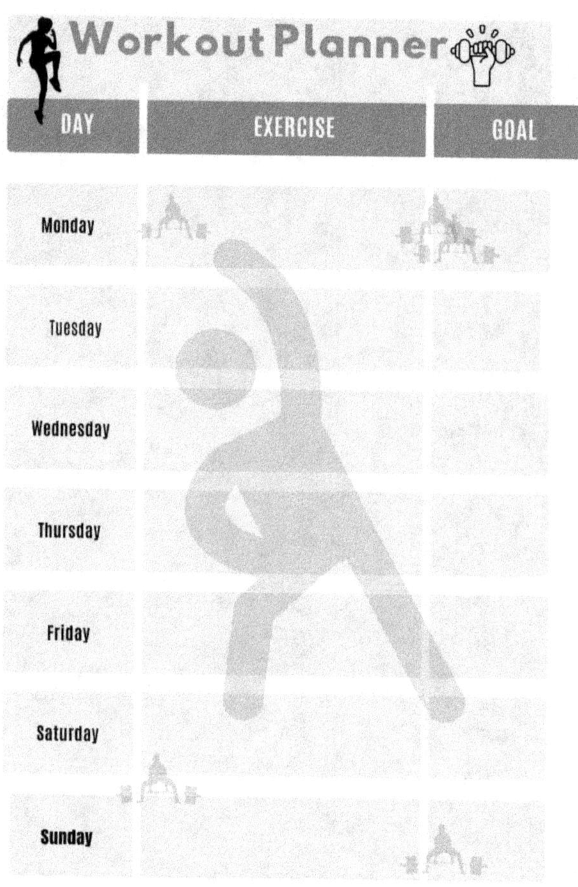

DAY	EXERCISE	GOAL
Monday		
Tuesday		
Wednesday		
Thursday		
Friday		
Saturday		
Sunday		

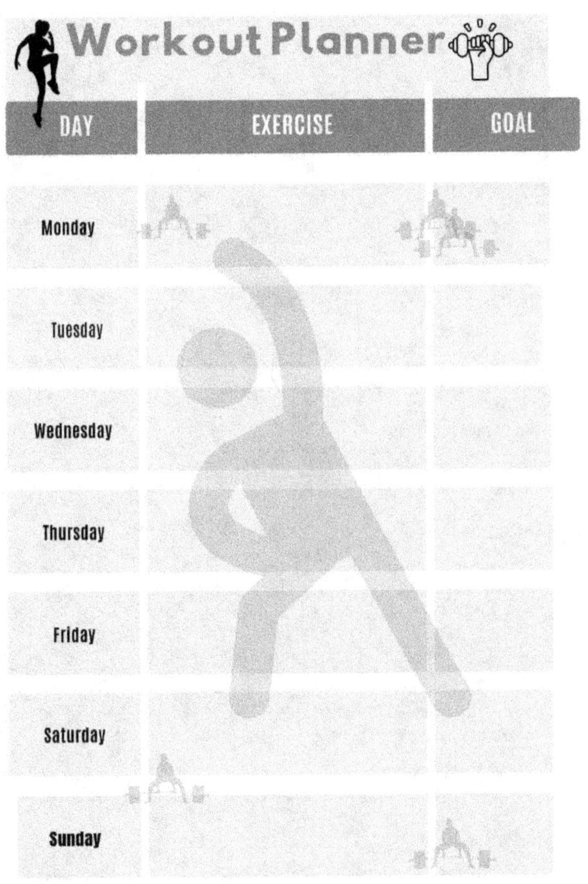

Workout Planner
DAY
EXERCISE
GOAL
Monday
Tuesday
Wednesday
Thursday
Friday
Saturday
Sunday

Workout Planner

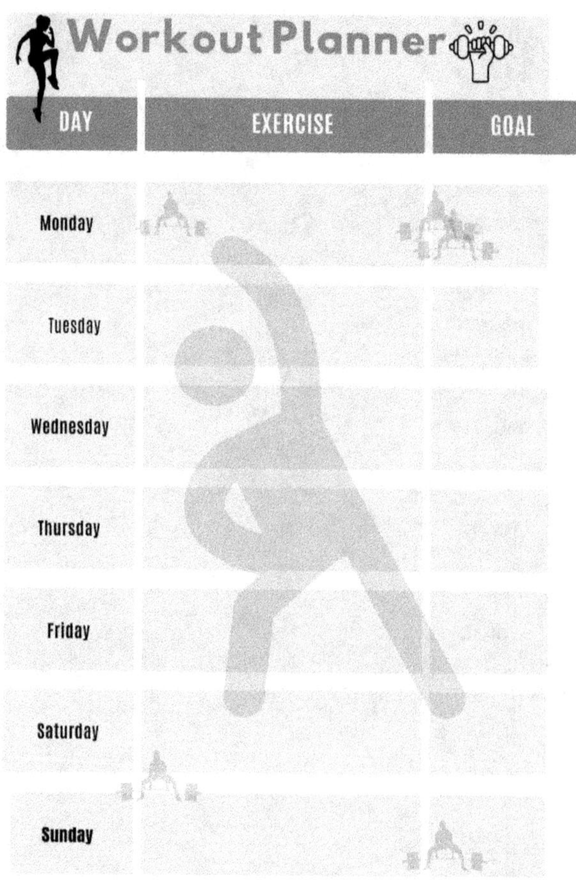

DAY	EXERCISE	GOAL
Monday		
Tuesday		
Wednesday		
Thursday		
Friday		
Saturday		
Sunday		

Workout Planner

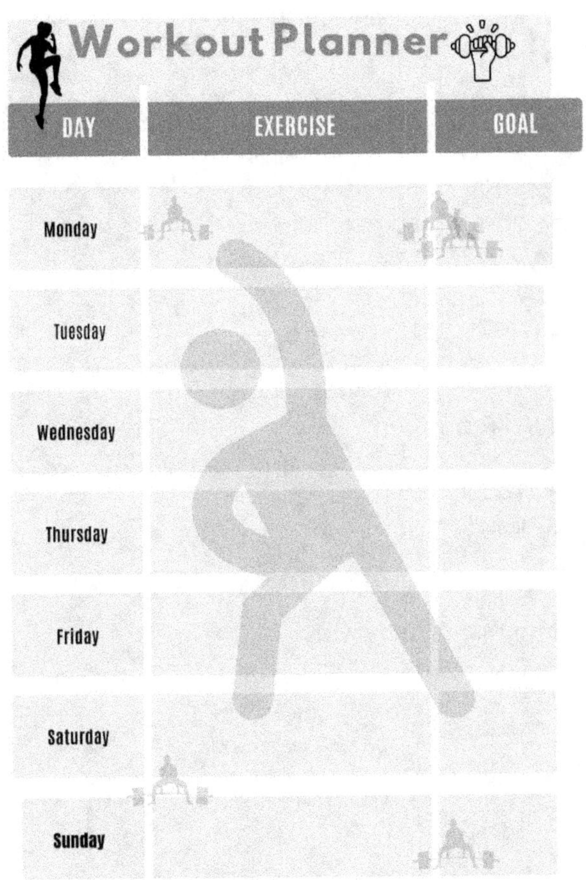

DAY	EXERCISE	GOAL
Monday		
Tuesday		
Wednesday		
Thursday		
Friday		
Saturday		
Sunday		

Workout Planner

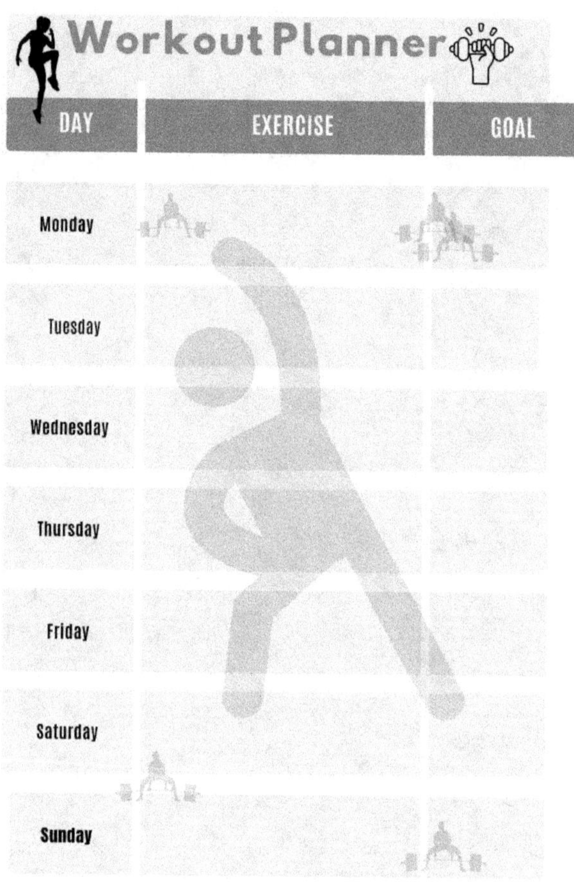

DAY	EXERCISE	GOAL
Monday		
Tuesday		
Wednesday		
Thursday		
Friday		
Saturday		
Sunday		

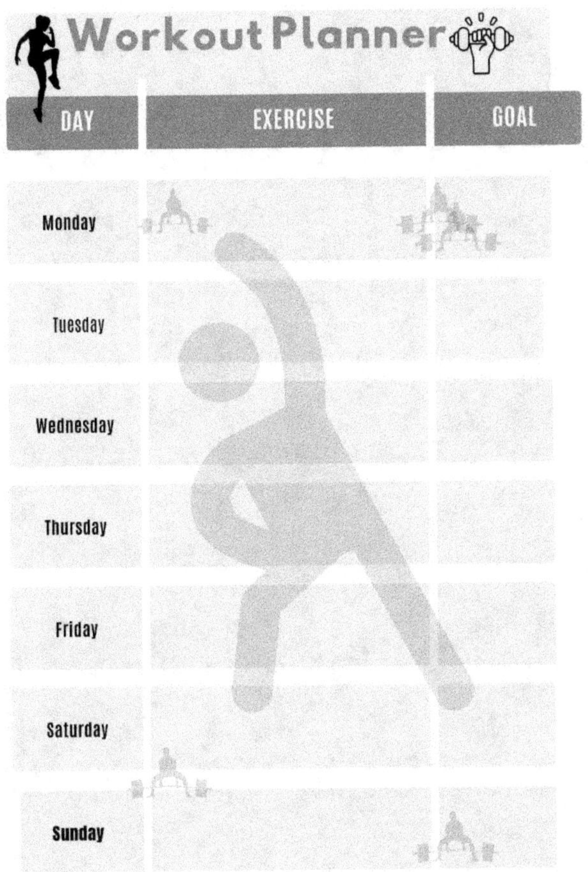

Workout Planner
DAY
EXERCISE
GOAL
Monday
Tuesday
Wednesday
Thursday
Friday
Saturday
Sunday

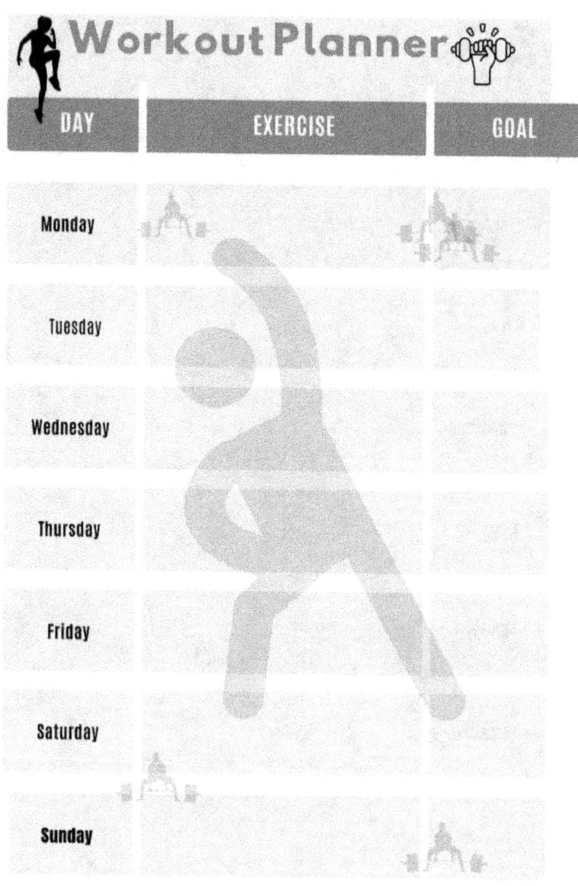

Workout Planner
DAY
EXERCISE
GOAL
Monday
Tuesday
Wednesday
Thursday
Friday
Saturday
Sunday

Workout Planner

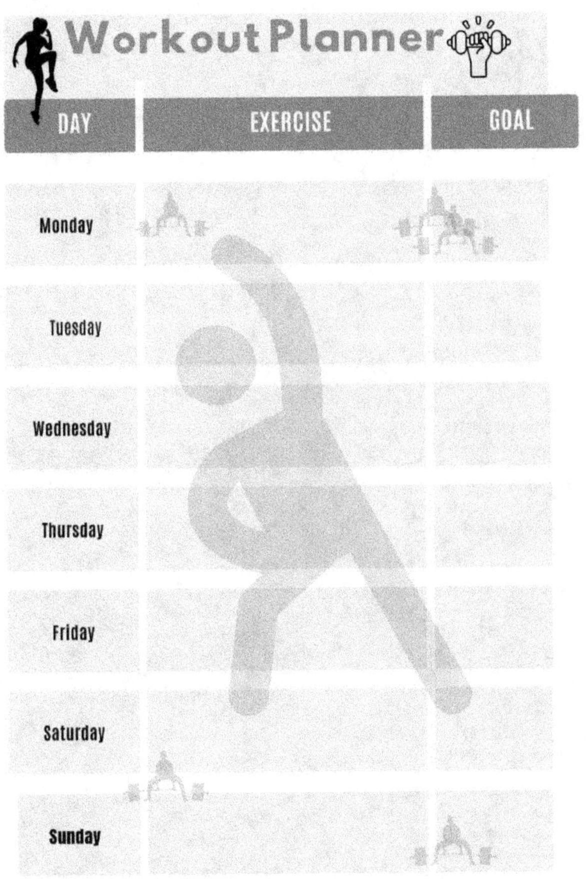

DAY	EXERCISE	GOAL
Monday		
Tuesday		
Wednesday		
Thursday		
Friday		
Saturday		
Sunday		

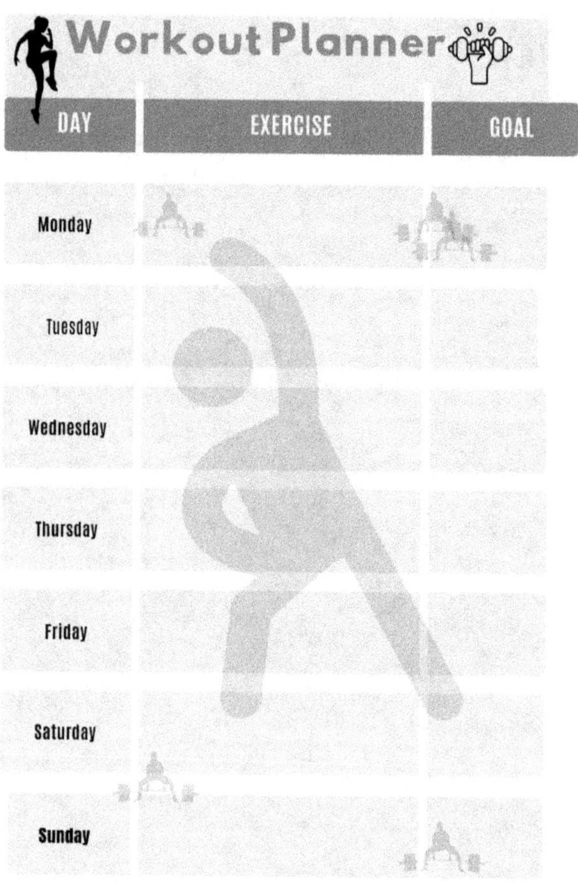

Workout Planner
DAY
EXERCISE
GOAL
Monday
Tuesday
Wednesday
Thursday
Friday
Saturday
Sunday

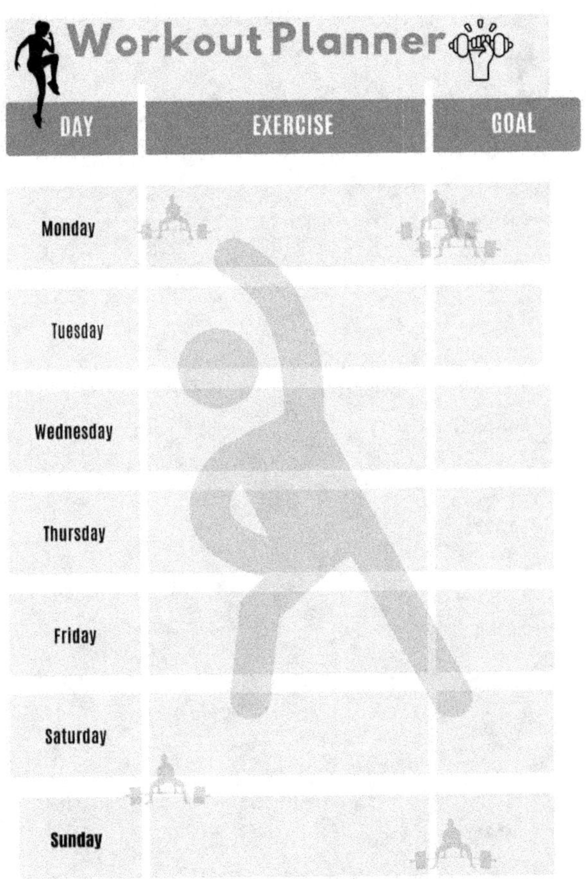
Workout Planner
DAY
EXERCISE
GOAL
Monday
Tuesday
Wednesday
Thursday
Friday
Saturday
Sunday

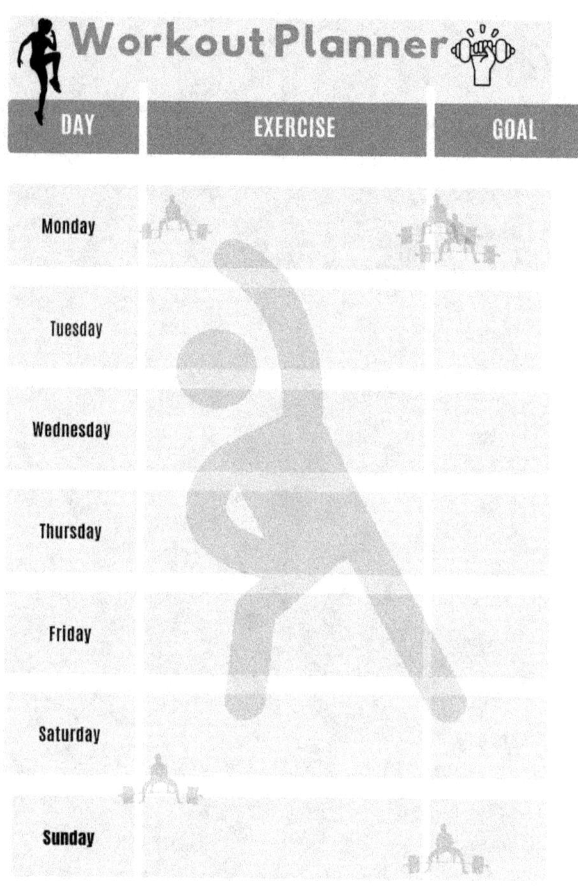

Workout Planner
DAY
EXERCISE
GOAL
Monday
Tuesday
Wednesday
Thursday
Friday
Saturday
Sunday

Workout Planner

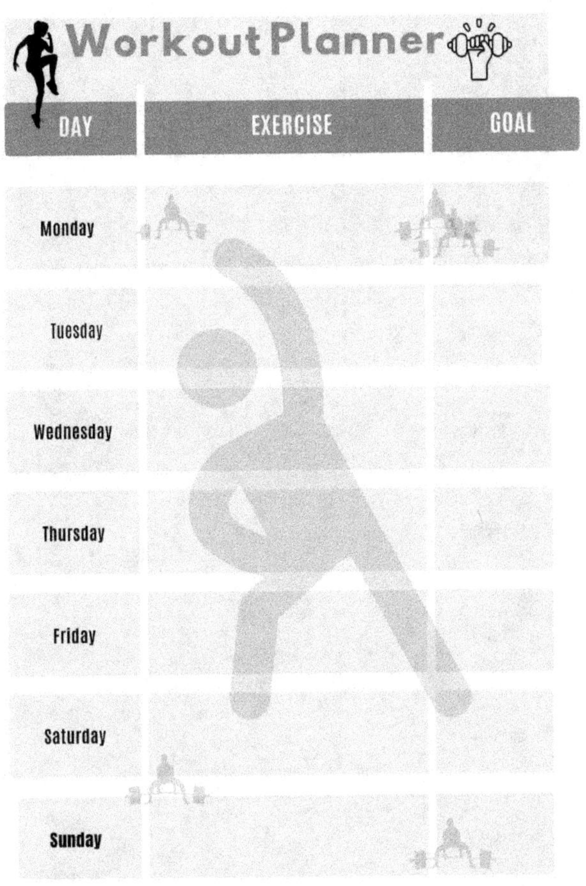

DAY	EXERCISE	GOAL
Monday		
Tuesday		
Wednesday		
Thursday		
Friday		
Saturday		
Sunday		

Workout Planner

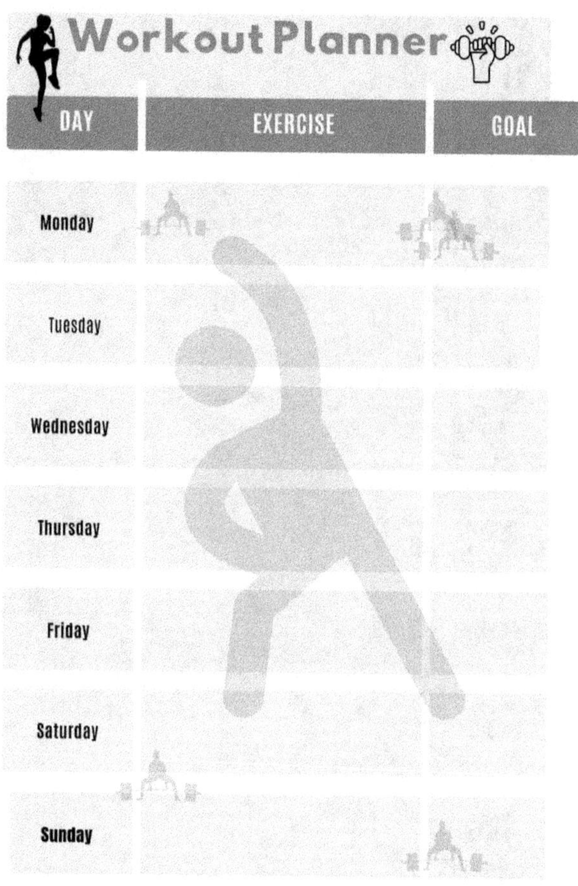

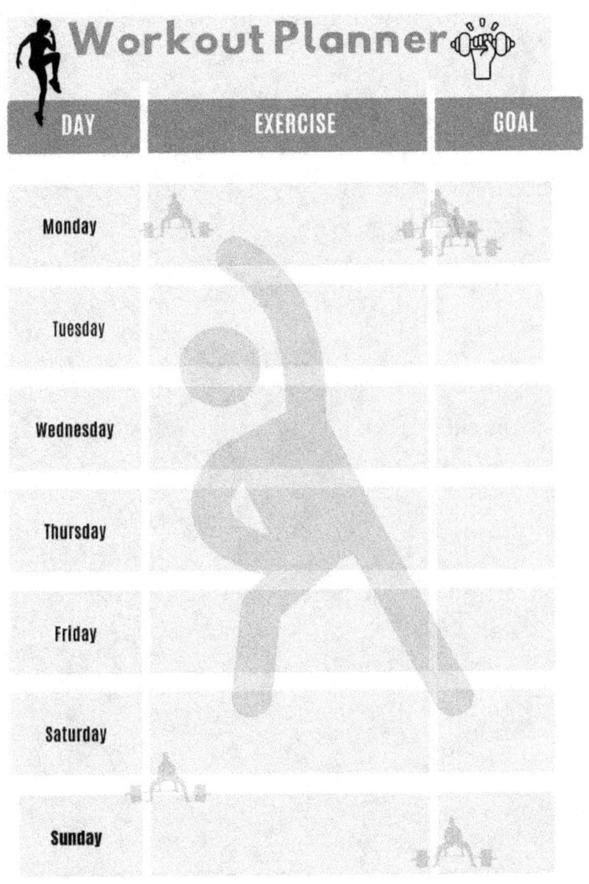

130

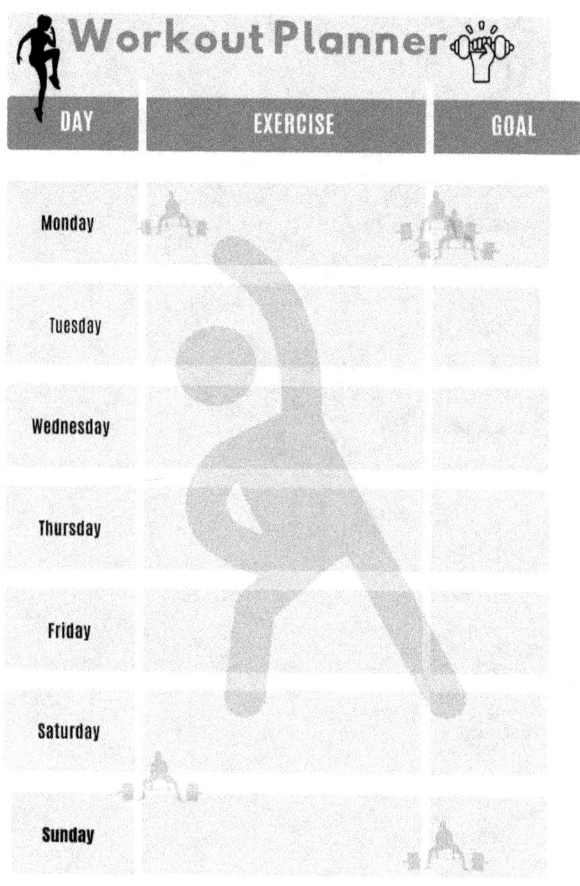
Workout Planner
DAY
EXERCISE
GOAL
Monday
Tuesday
Wednesday
Thursday
Friday
Saturday
Sunday

Workout Planner

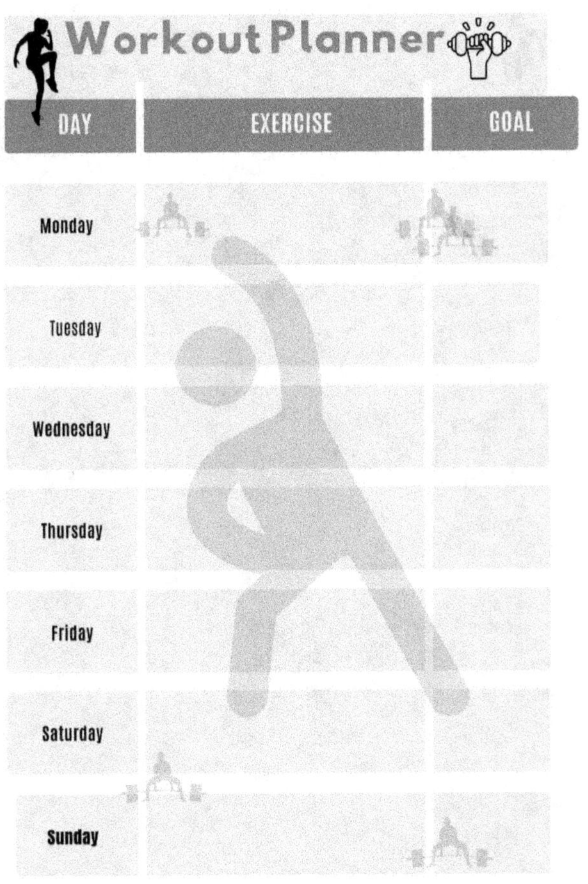

DAY	EXERCISE	GOAL
Monday		
Tuesday		
Wednesday		
Thursday		
Friday		
Saturday		
Sunday		

Workout Planner

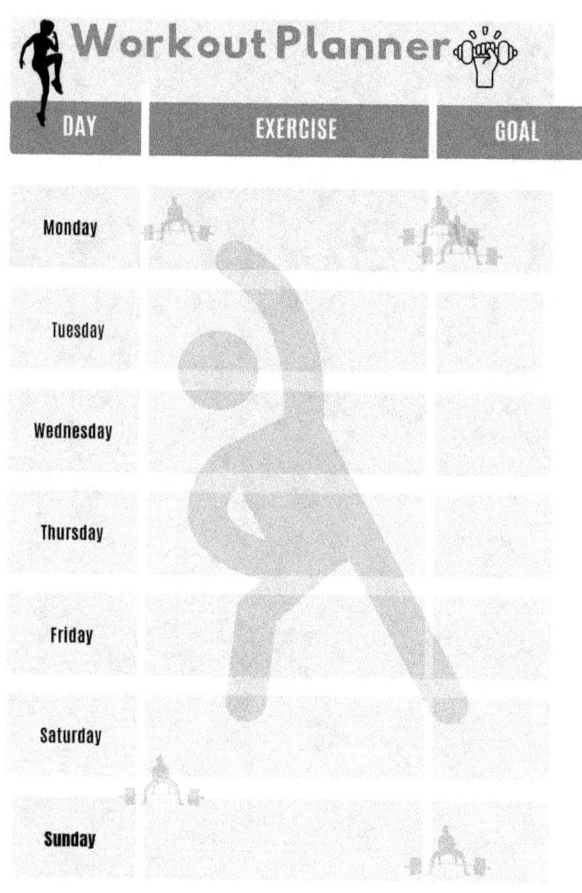

DAY	EXERCISE	GOAL
Monday		
Tuesday		
Wednesday		
Thursday		
Friday		
Saturday		
Sunday		

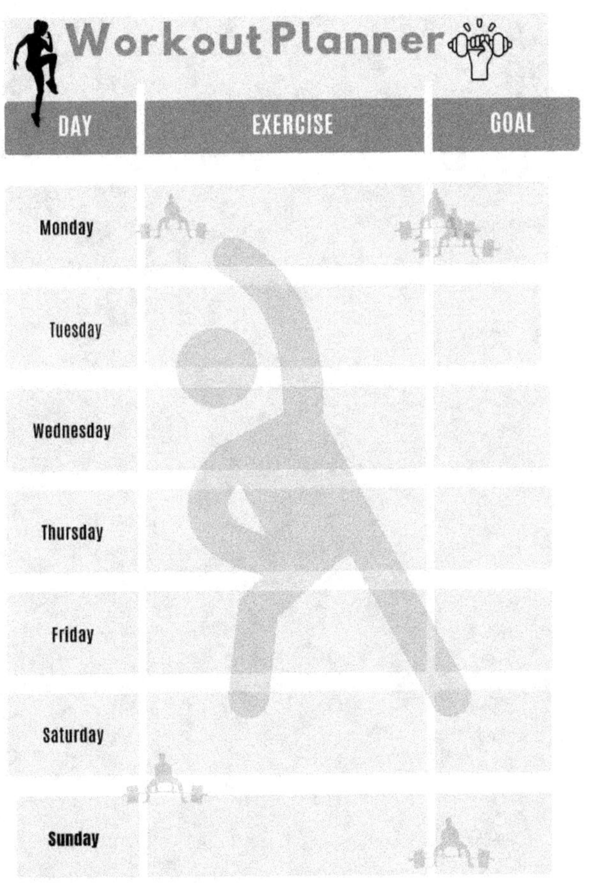

Workout Planner
DAY
EXERCISE
GOAL
Monday
Tuesday
Wednesday
Thursday
Friday
Saturday
Sunday

Workout Planner

DAY	EXERCISE	GOAL
Monday		
Tuesday		
Wednesday		
Thursday		
Friday		
Saturday		
Sunday		

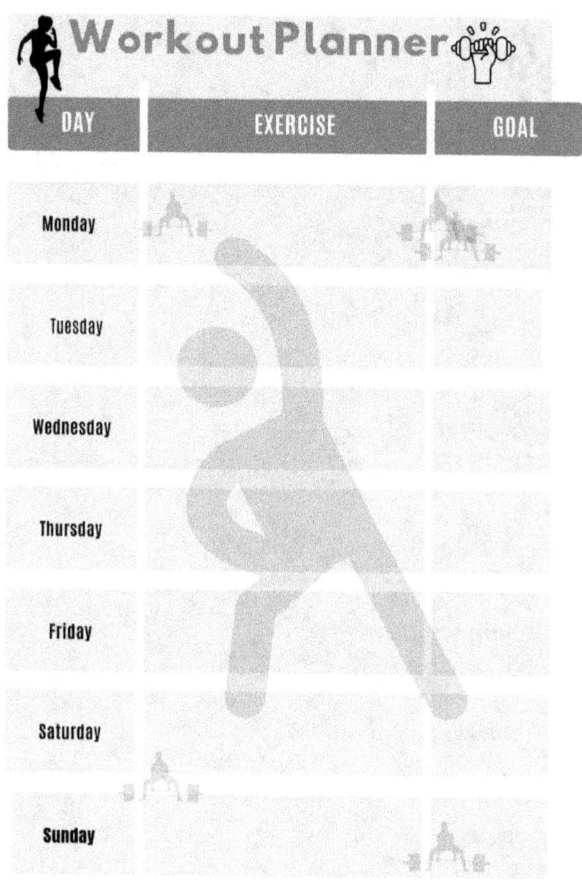

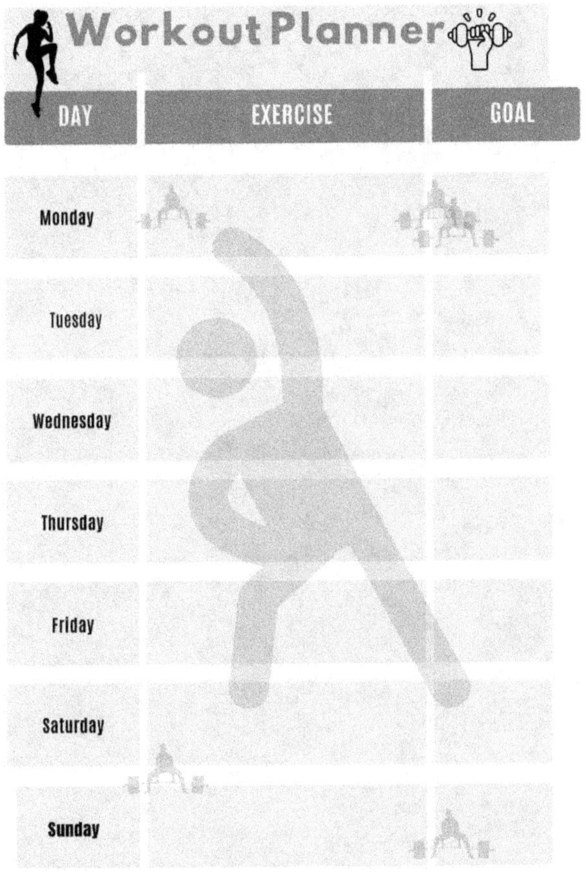

Workout Planner
DAY
EXERCISE
GOAL
Monday
Tuesday
Wednesday
Thursday
Friday
Saturday
Sunday

Workout Planner

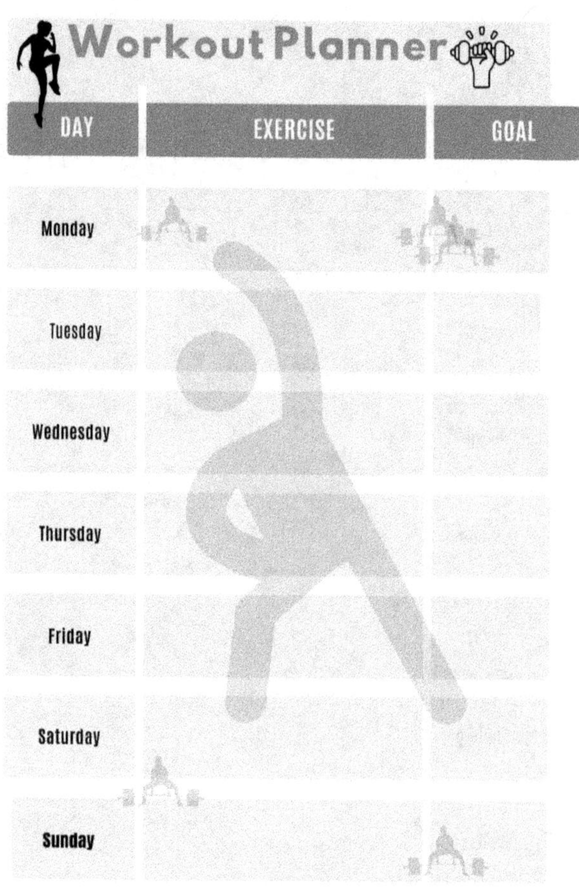

DAY	EXERCISE	GOAL
Monday		
Tuesday		
Wednesday		
Thursday		
Friday		
Saturday		
Sunday		

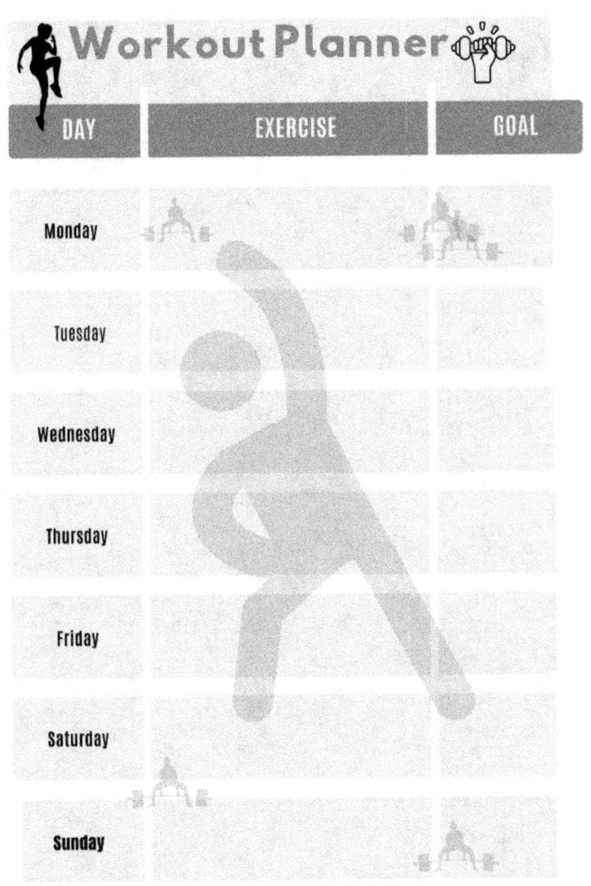

Workout Planner
DAY
EXERCISE
GOAL
Monday
Tuesday
Wednesday
Thursday
Friday
Saturday
Sunday

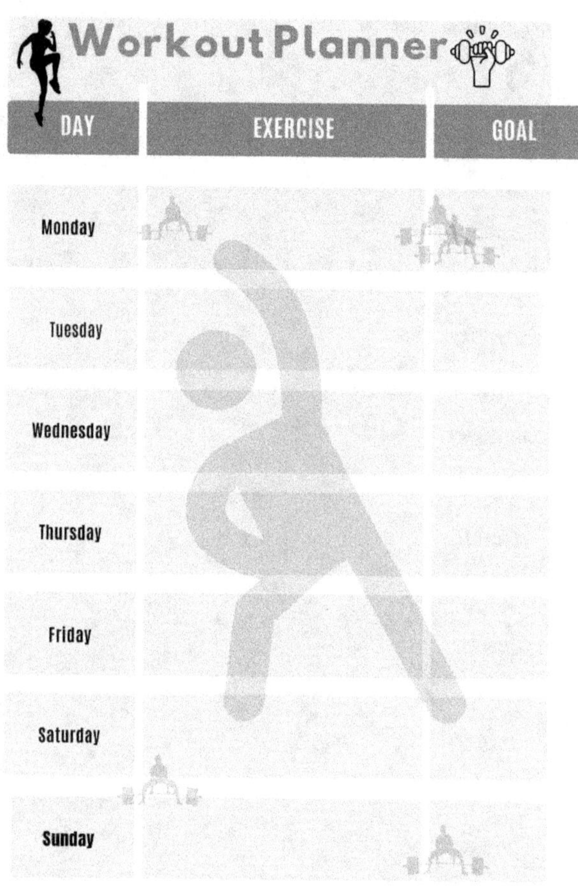

Workout Planner
DAY
EXERCISE
GOAL
Monday
Tuesday
Wednesday
Thursday
Friday
Saturday
Sunday

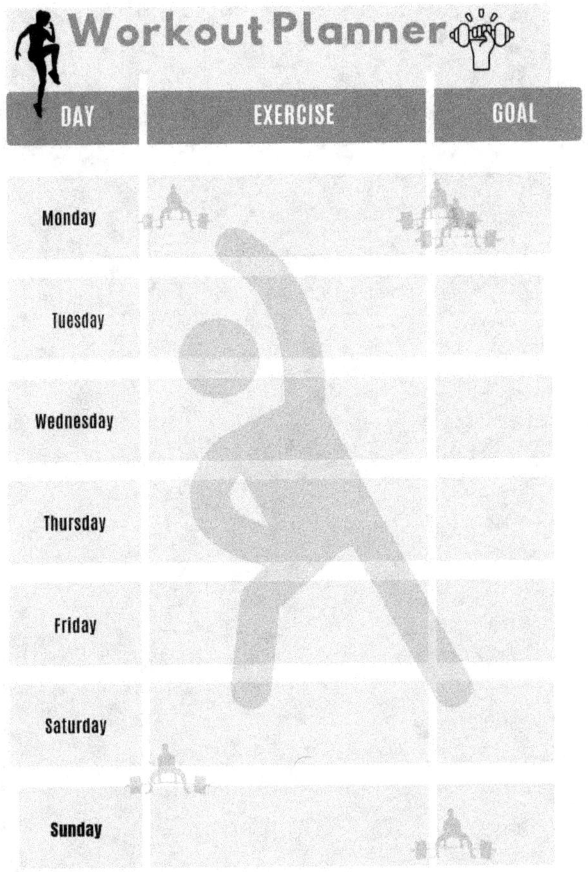

Workout Planner
DAY
EXERCISE
GOAL
Monday
Tuesday
Wednesday
Thursday
Friday
Saturday
Sunday

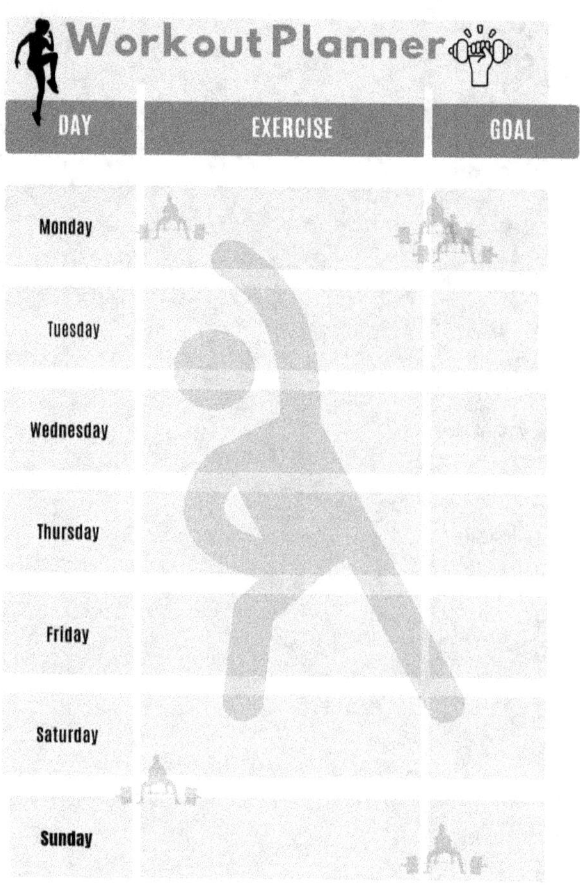

Workout Planner
DAY
EXERCISE
GOAL
Monday
Tuesday
Wednesday
Thursday
Friday
Saturday
Sunday

Workout Planner

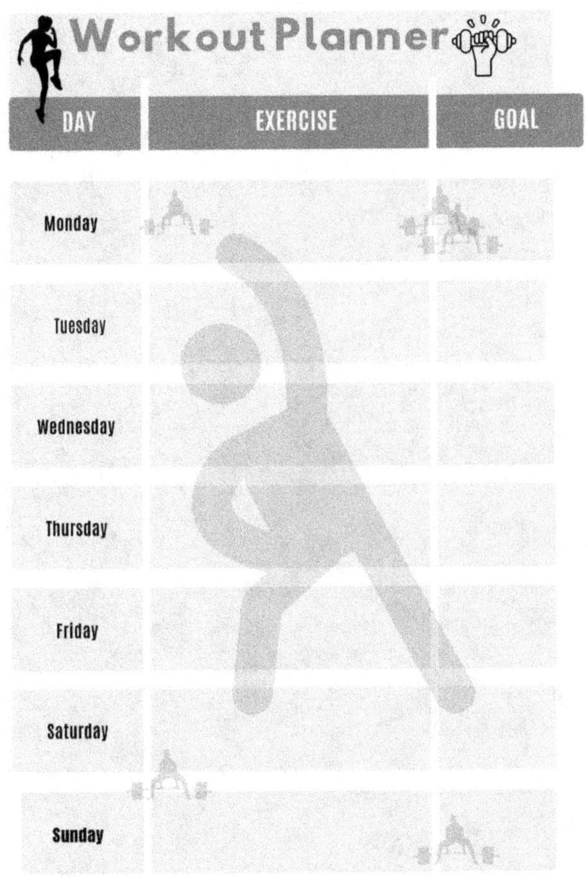

DAY	EXERCISE	GOAL
Monday		
Tuesday		
Wednesday		
Thursday		
Friday		
Saturday		
Sunday		

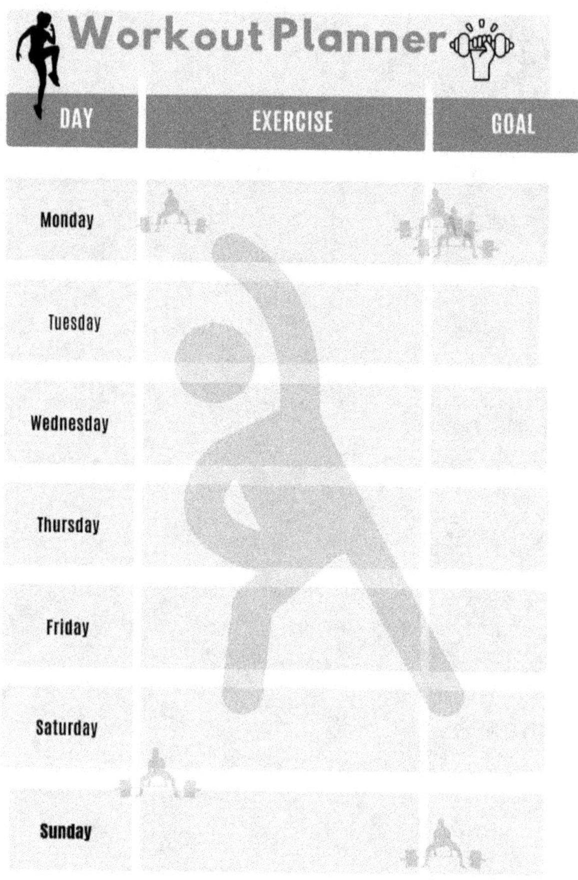
Workout Planner
DAY
EXERCISE
GOAL
Monday
Tuesday
Wednesday
Thursday
Friday
Saturday
Sunday

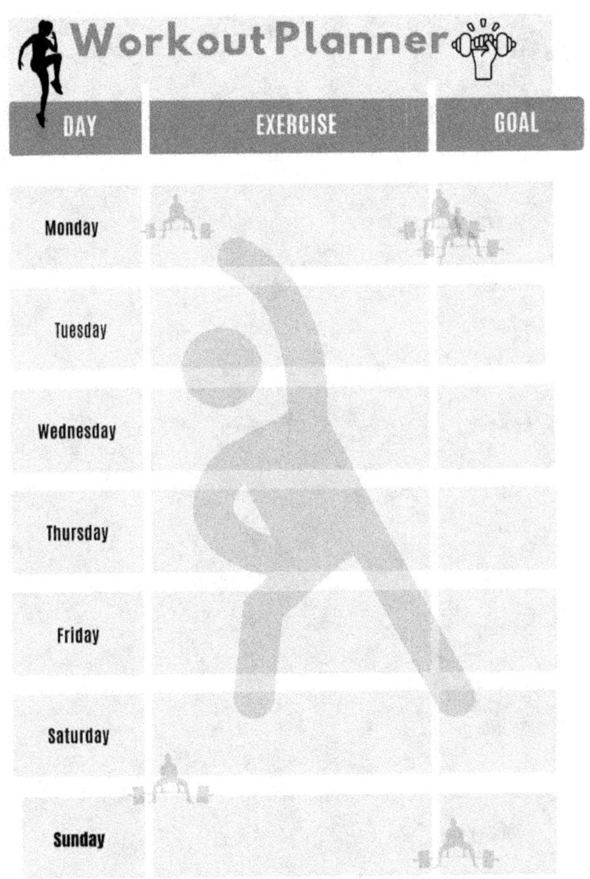

Workout Planner
DAY
EXERCISE
GOAL
Monday
Tuesday
Wednesday
Thursday
Friday
Saturday
Sunday

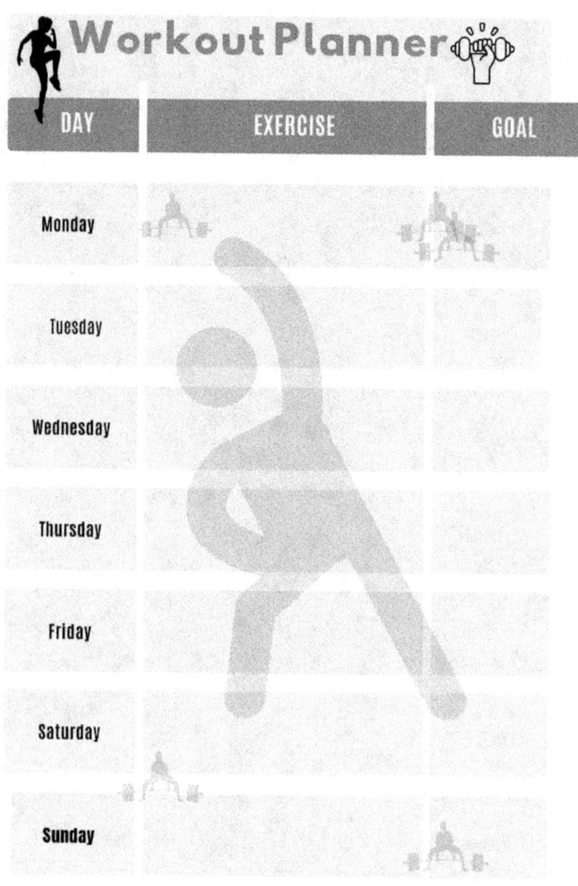

Workout Planner
DAY
EXERCISE
GOAL
Monday
Tuesday
Wednesday
Thursday
Friday
Saturday
Sunday

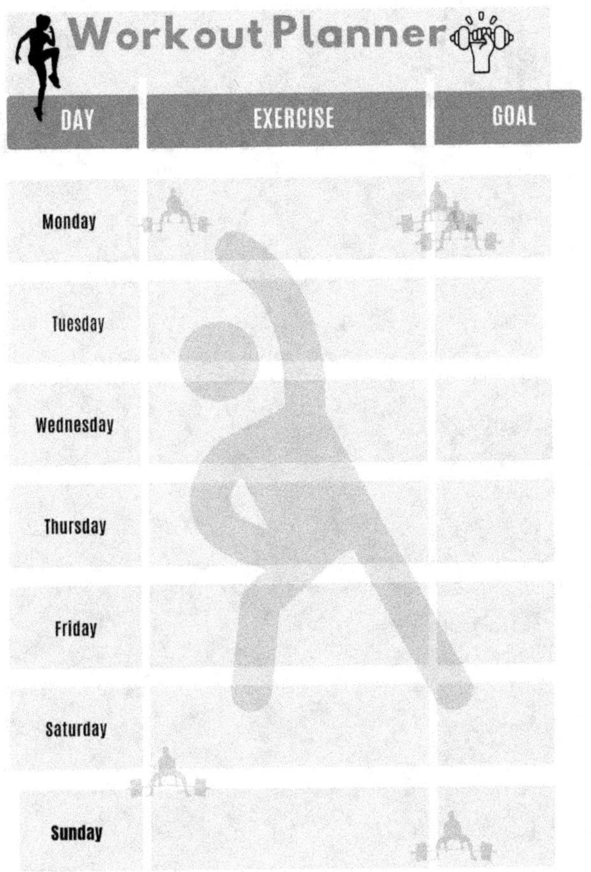

Workout Planner
DAY
EXERCISE
GOAL
Monday
Tuesday
Wednesday
Thursday
Friday
Saturday
Sunday

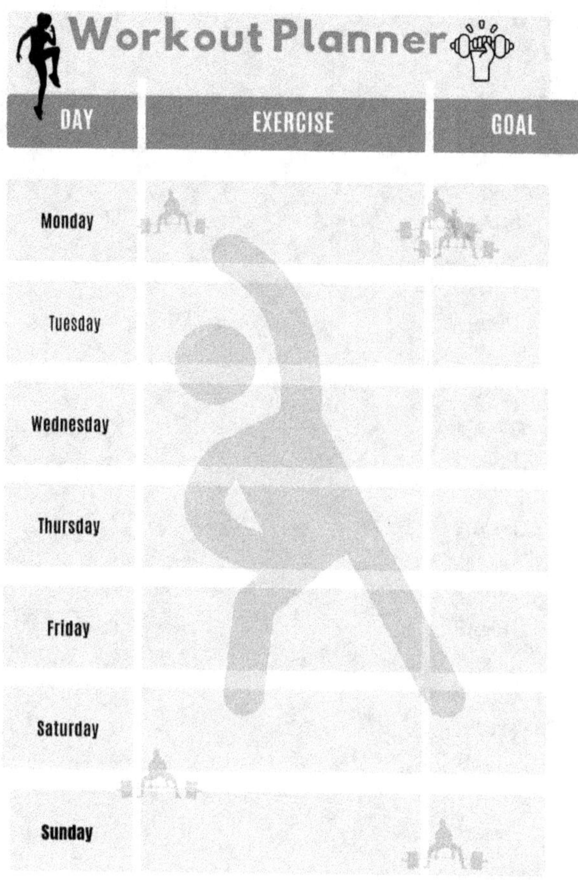

Workout Planner
DAY
EXERCISE
GOAL
Monday
Tuesday
Wednesday
Thursday
Friday
Saturday
Sunday

Workout Planner

DAY	EXERCISE	GOAL
Monday		
Tuesday		
Wednesday		
Thursday		
Friday		
Saturday		
Sunday		

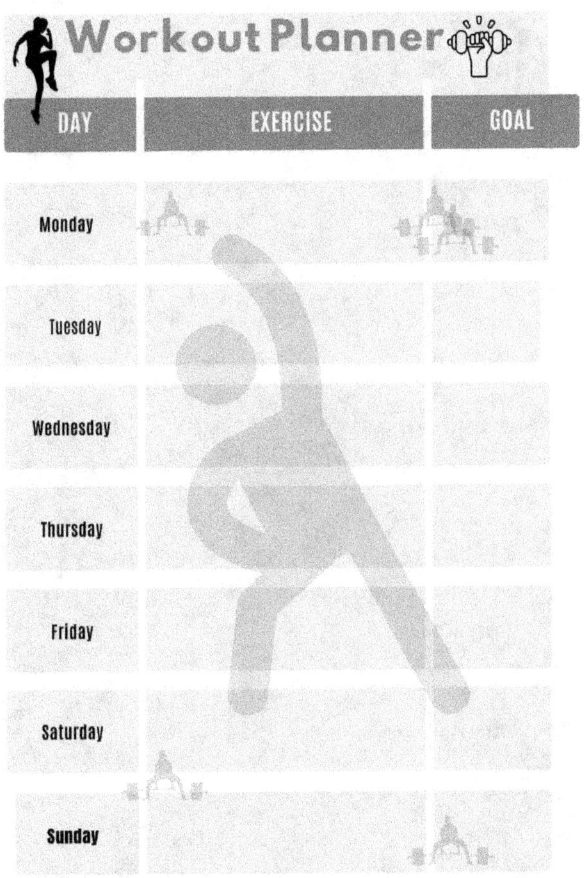

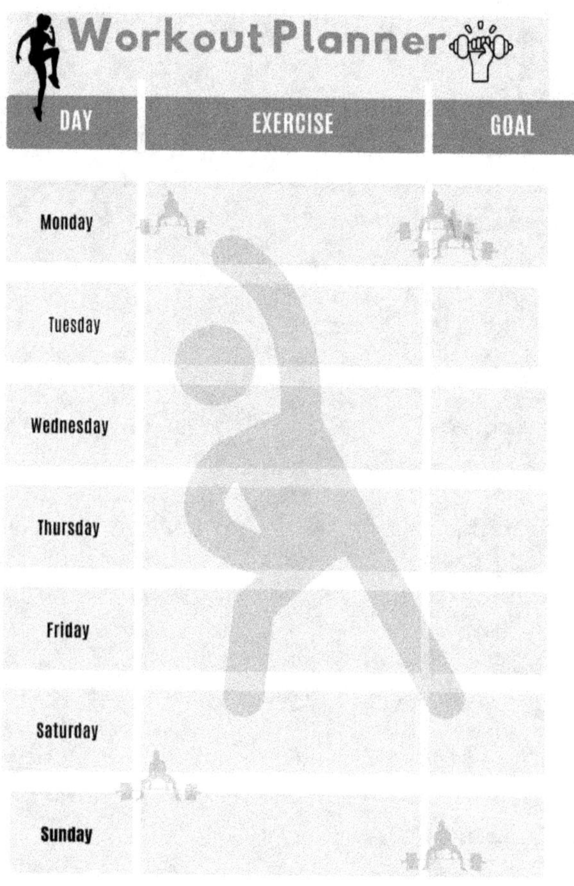
Workout Planner
DAY
EXERCISE
GOAL
Monday
Tuesday
Wednesday
Thursday
Friday
Saturday
Sunday

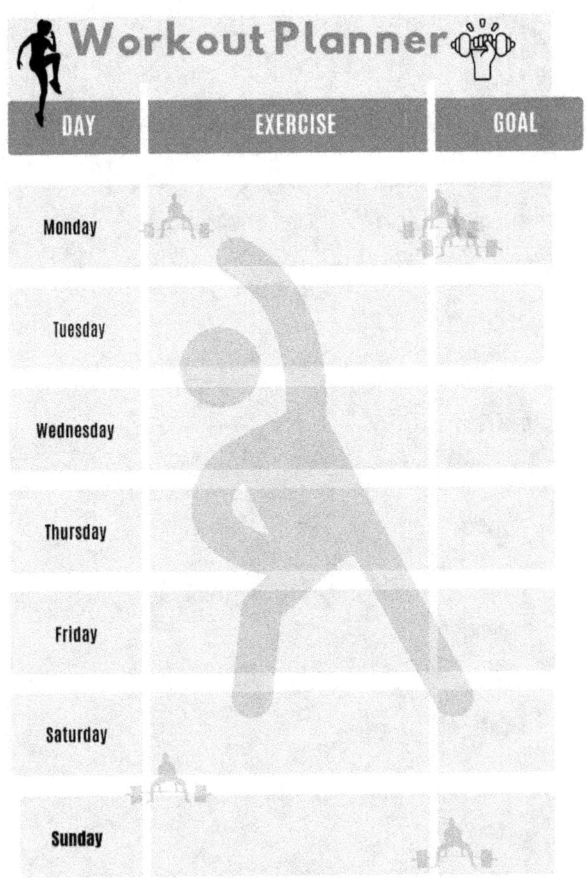

Workout Planner
DAY
EXERCISE
GOAL
Monday
Tuesday
Wednesday
Thursday
Friday
Saturday
Sunday

Workout Planner

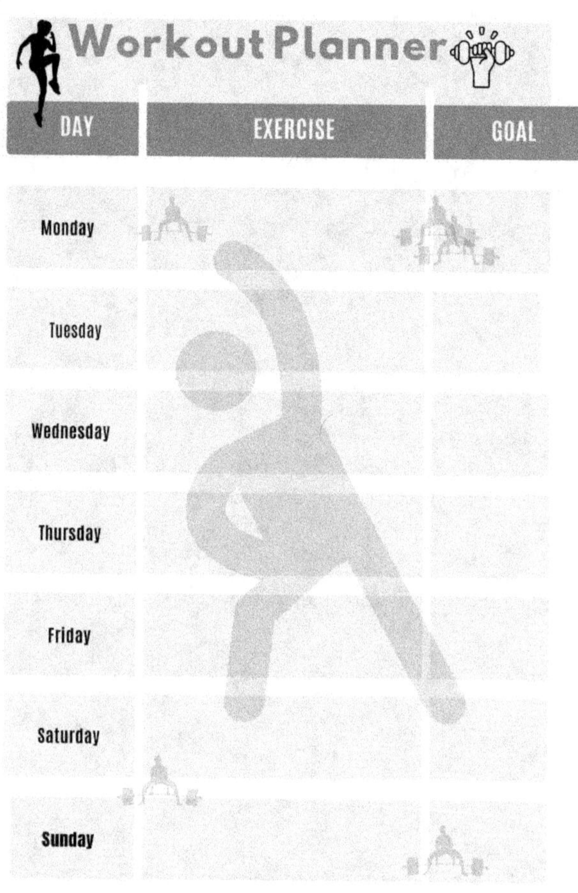

DAY	EXERCISE	GOAL
Monday		
Tuesday		
Wednesday		
Thursday		
Friday		
Saturday		
Sunday		

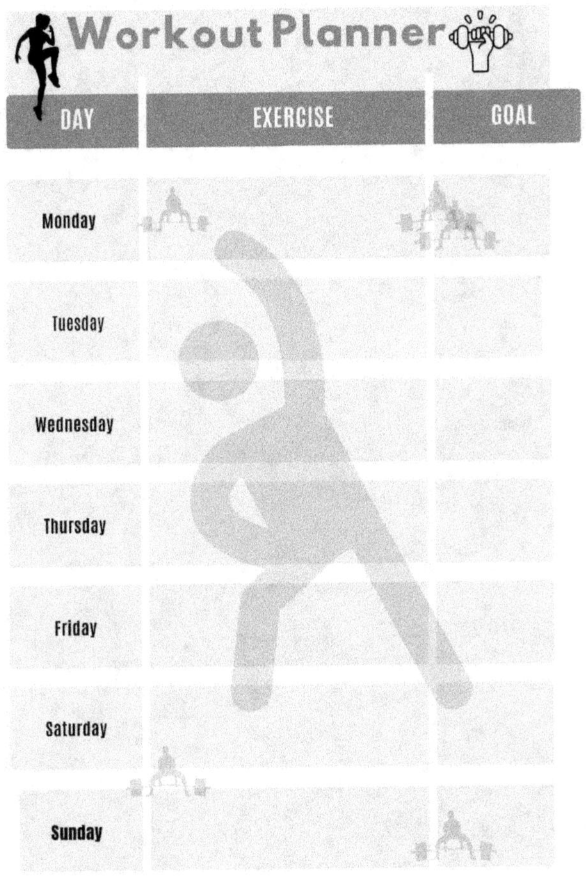

Workout Planner
DAY
EXERCISE
GOAL
Monday
Tuesday
Wednesday
Thursday
Friday
Saturday
Sunday

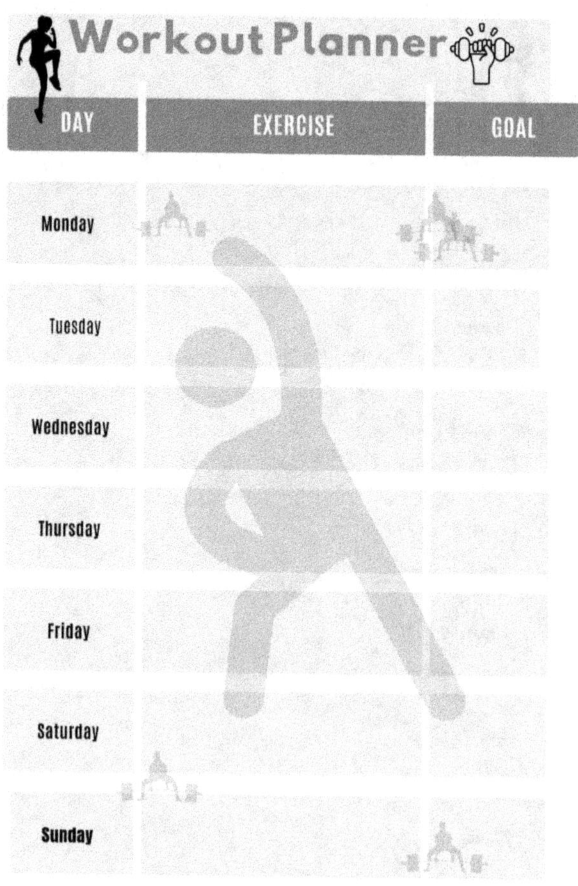

Workout Planner
DAY
EXERCISE
GOAL
Monday
Tuesday
Wednesday
Thursday
Friday
Saturday
Sunday

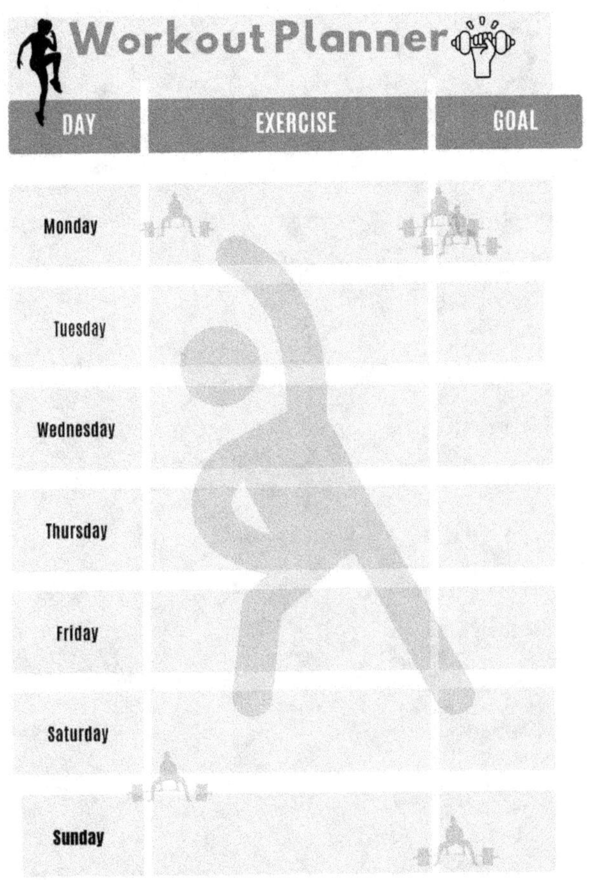

Workout Planner
DAY
EXERCISE
GOAL
Monday
Tuesday
Wednesday
Thursday
Friday
Saturday
Sunday

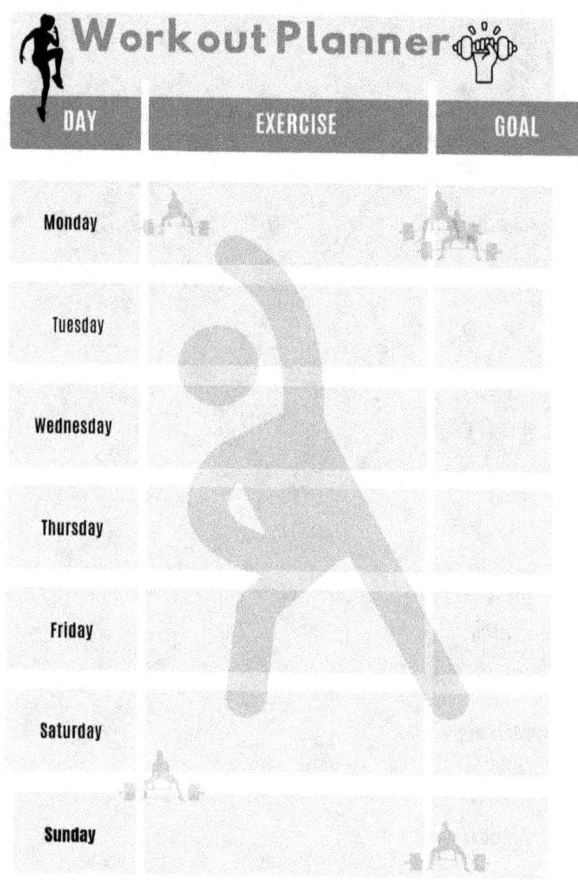

Workout Planner
DAY
EXERCISE
GOAL
Monday
Tuesday
Wednesday
Thursday
Friday
Saturday
Sunday

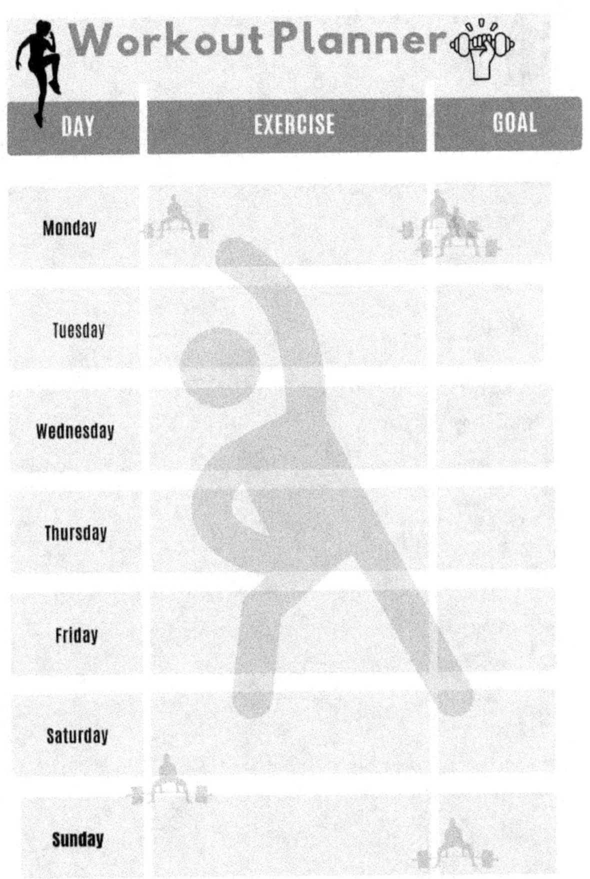
Workout Planner
DAY
EXERCISE
GOAL
Monday
Tuesday
Wednesday
Thursday
Friday
Saturday
Sunday

Workout Planner

DAY	EXERCISE	GOAL
Monday		
Tuesday		
Wednesday		
Thursday		
Friday		
Saturday		
Sunday		

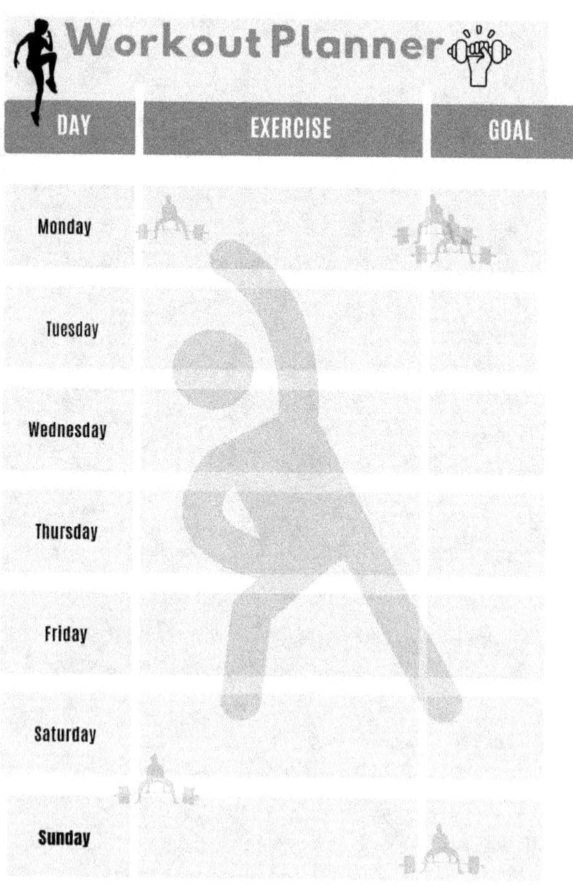

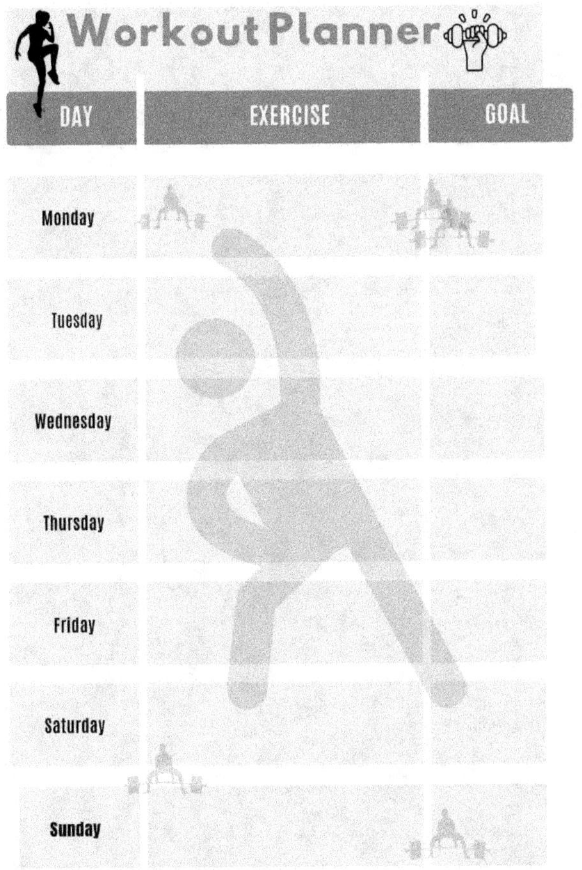

Workout Planner
DAY
EXERCISE
GOAL
Monday
Tuesday
Wednesday
Thursday
Friday
Saturday
Sunday

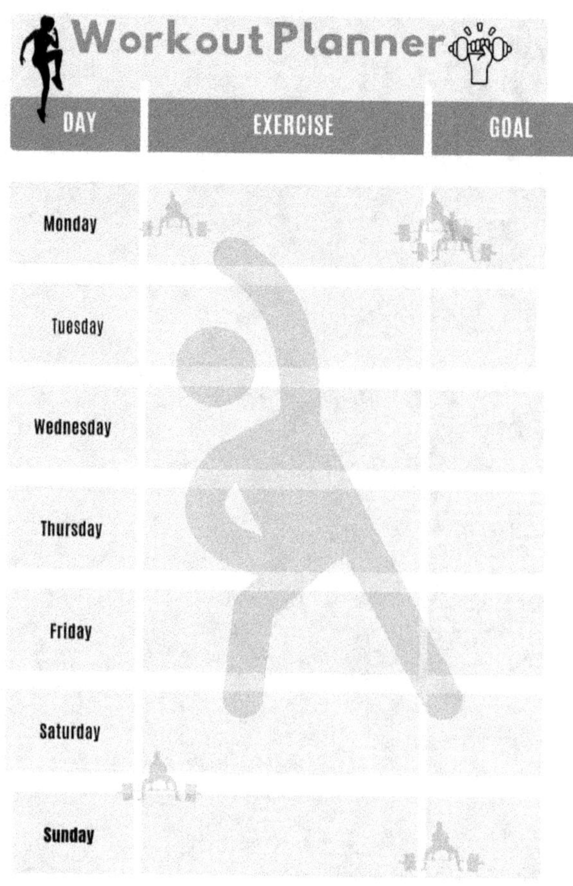

Workout Planner
DAY
EXERCISE
GOAL
Monday
Tuesday
Wednesday
Thursday
Friday
Saturday
Sunday

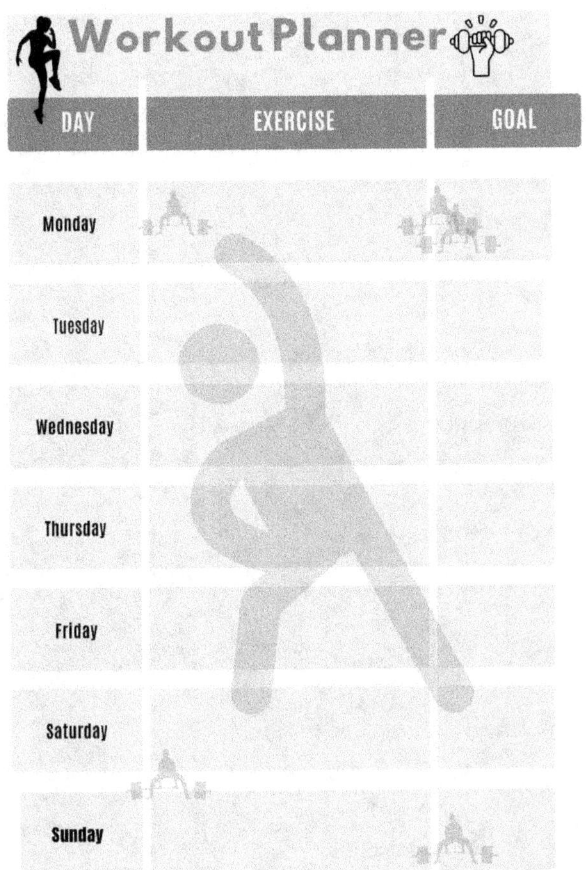

Workout Planner
DAY
EXERCISE
GOAL
Monday
Tuesday
Wednesday
Thursday
Friday
Saturday
Sunday

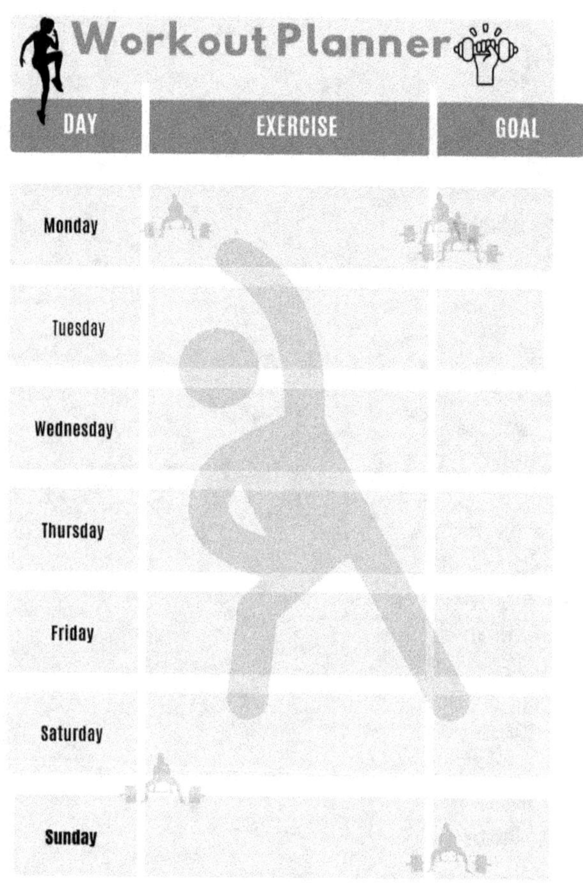
Workout Planner
DAY
EXERCISE
GOAL
Monday
Tuesday
Wednesday
Thursday
Friday
Saturday
Sunday

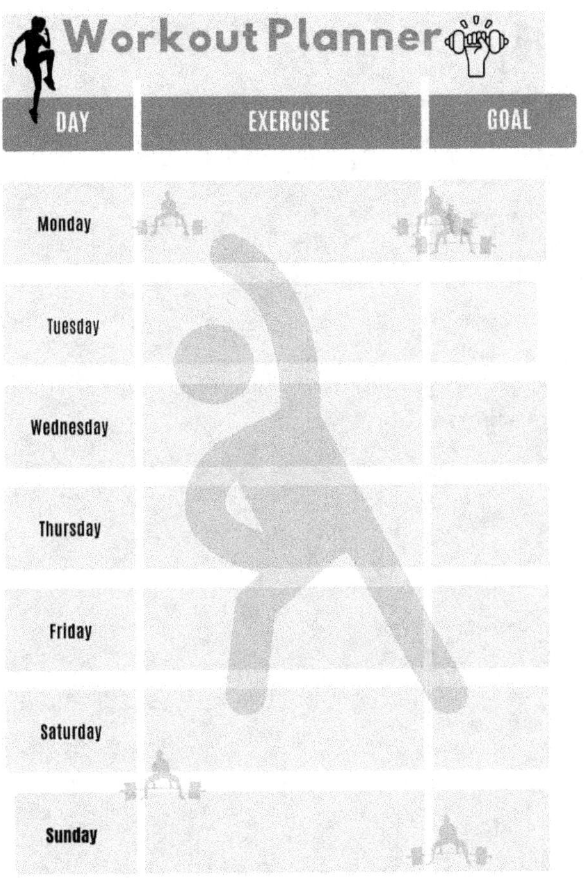

Workout Planner
DAY
EXERCISE
GOAL
Monday
Tuesday
Wednesday
Thursday
Friday
Saturday
Sunday

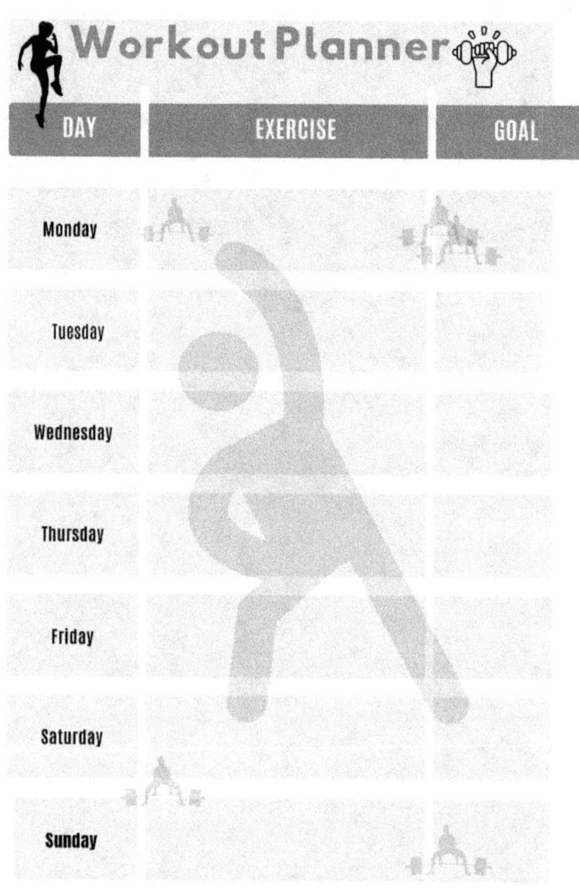

Workout Planner
DAY
EXERCISE
GOAL
Monday
Tuesday
Wednesday
Thursday
Friday
Saturday
Sunday

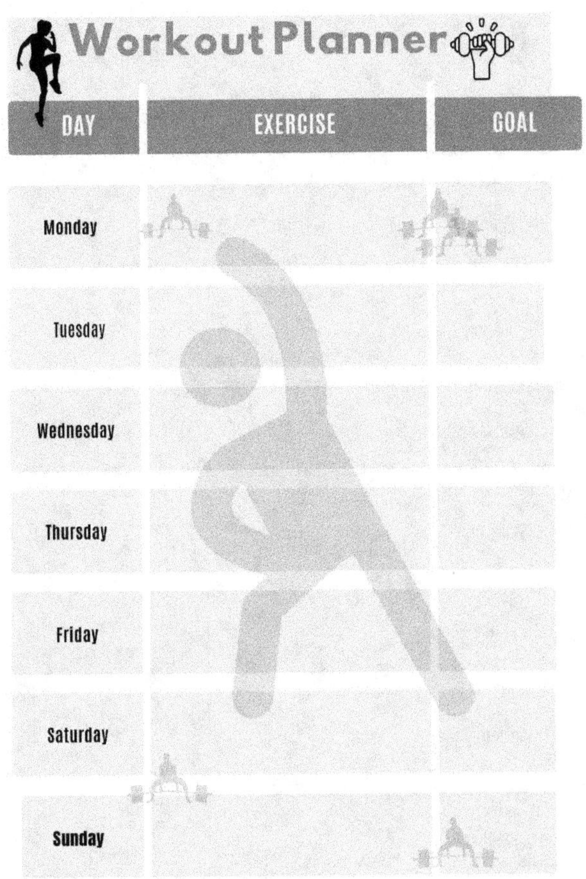

DAY	EXERCISE	GOAL
Monday		
Tuesday		
Wednesday		
Thursday		
Friday		
Saturday		
Sunday		

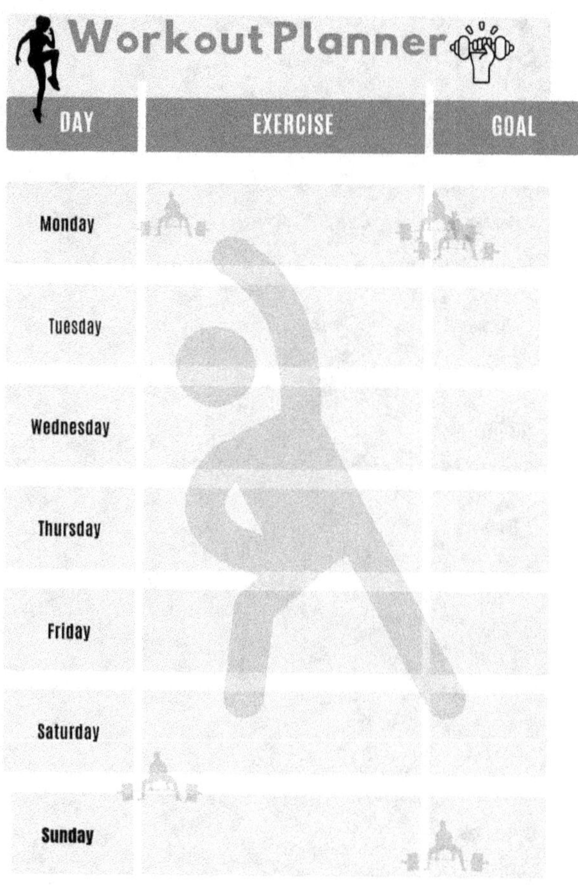
Workout Planner
DAY
EXERCISE
GOAL
Monday
Tuesday
Wednesday
Thursday
Friday
Saturday
Sunday

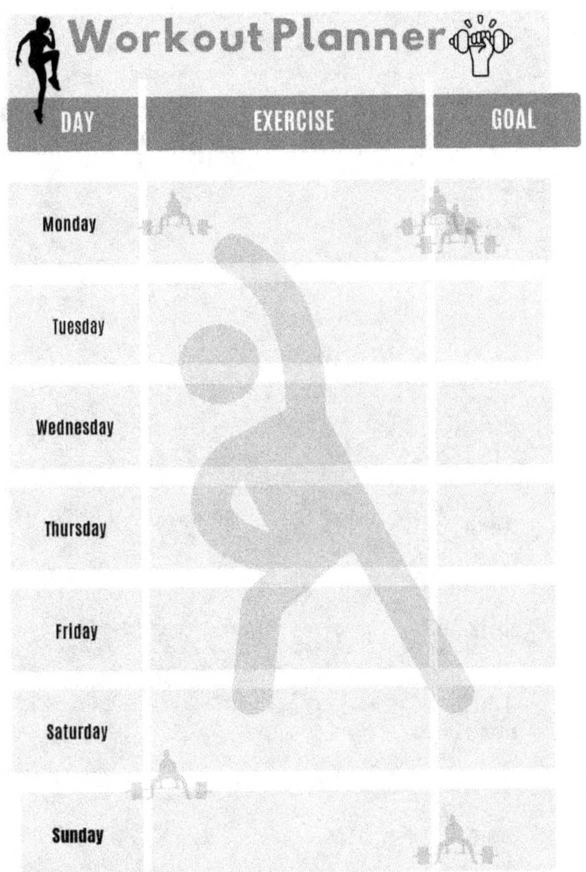

Workout Planner
DAY
EXERCISE
GOAL
Monday
Tuesday
Wednesday
Thursday
Friday
Saturday
Sunday

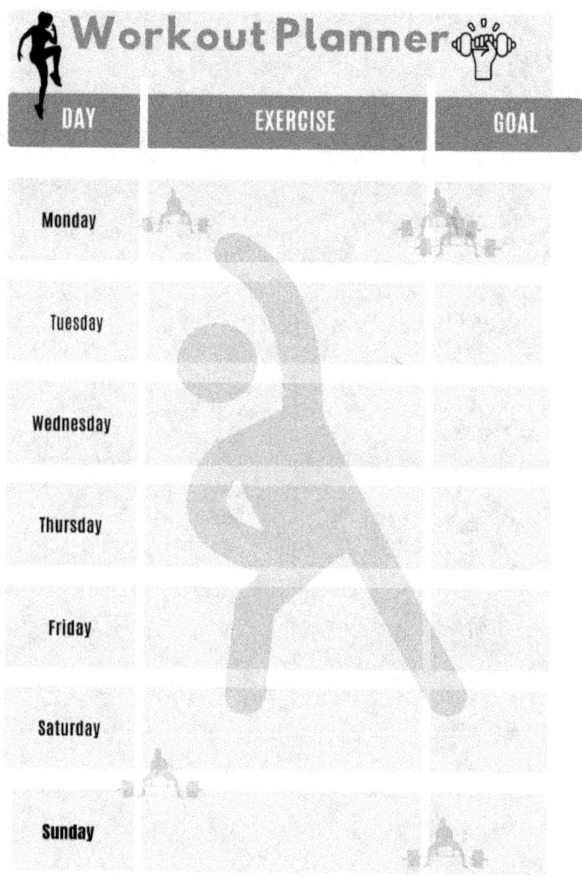
Workout Planner
DAY
EXERCISE
GOAL
Monday
Tuesday
Wednesday
Thursday
Friday
Saturday
Sunday

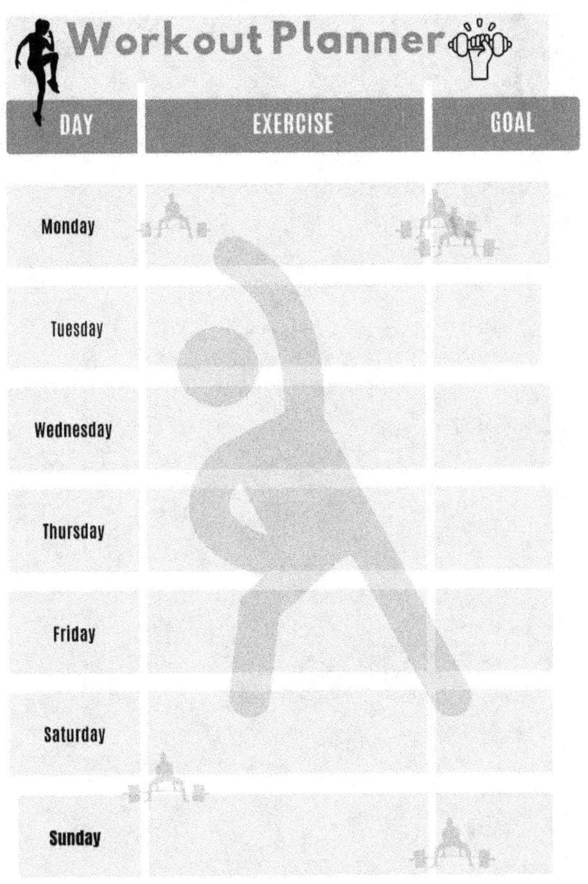

Workout Planner
DAY
EXERCISE
GOAL
Monday
Tuesday
Wednesday
Thursday
Friday
Saturday
Sunday

Workout Planner

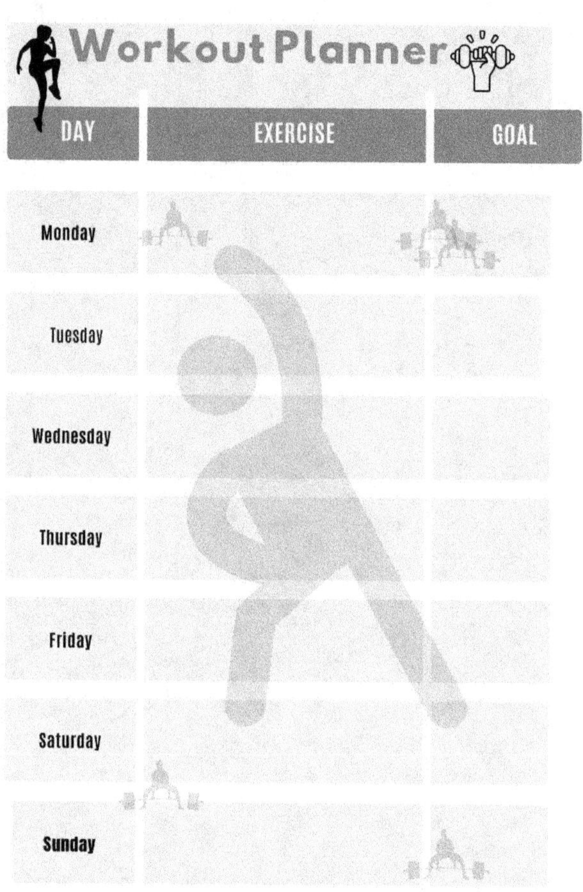

DAY	EXERCISE	GOAL
Monday		
Tuesday		
Wednesday		
Thursday		
Friday		
Saturday		
Sunday		

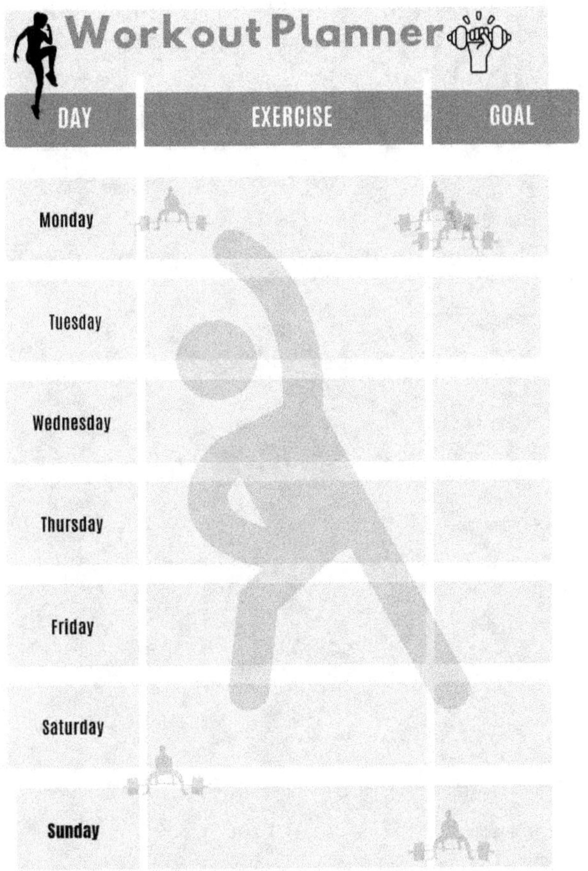

Workout Planner
DAY
EXERCISE
GOAL
Monday
Tuesday
Wednesday
Thursday
Friday
Saturday
Sunday

Workout Planner

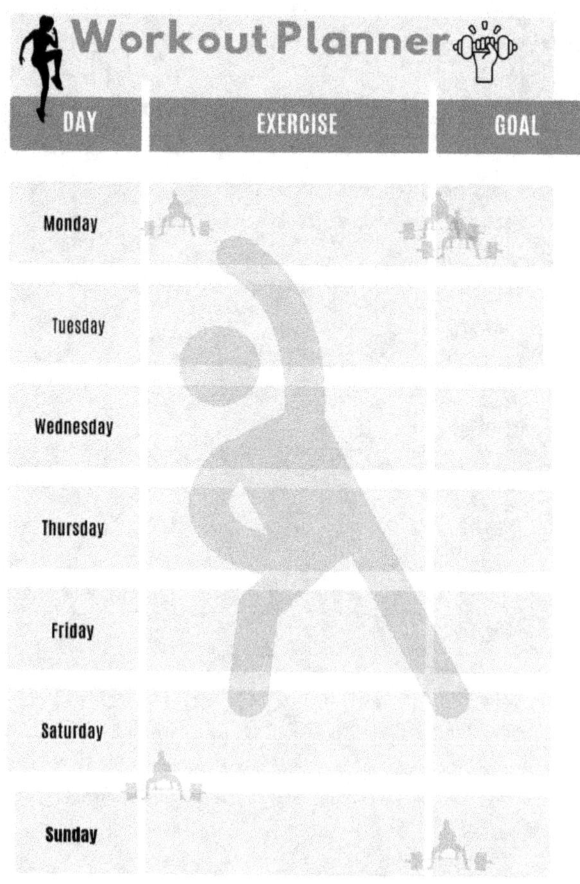

DAY	EXERCISE	GOAL
Monday		
Tuesday		
Wednesday		
Thursday		
Friday		
Saturday		
Sunday		

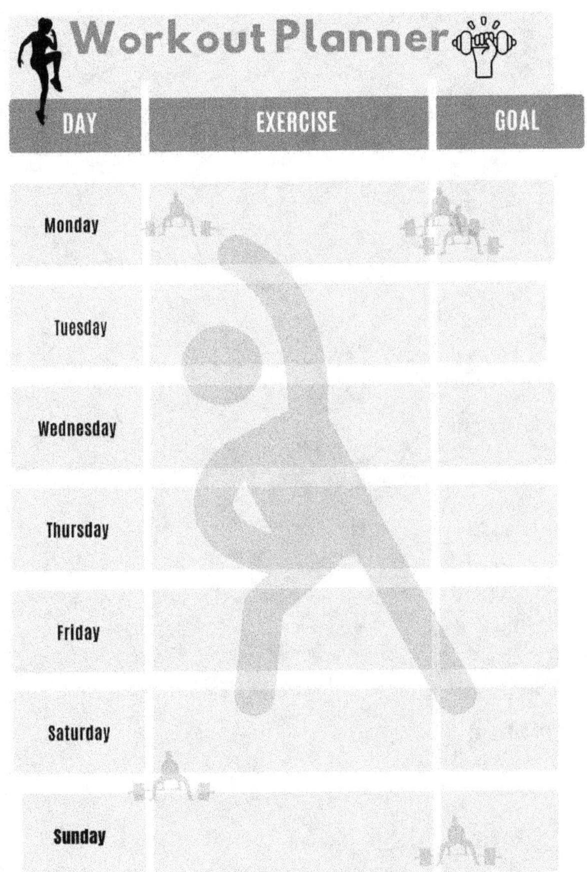

Workout Planner
DAY
EXERCISE
GOAL
Monday
Tuesday
Wednesday
Thursday
Friday
Saturday
Sunday

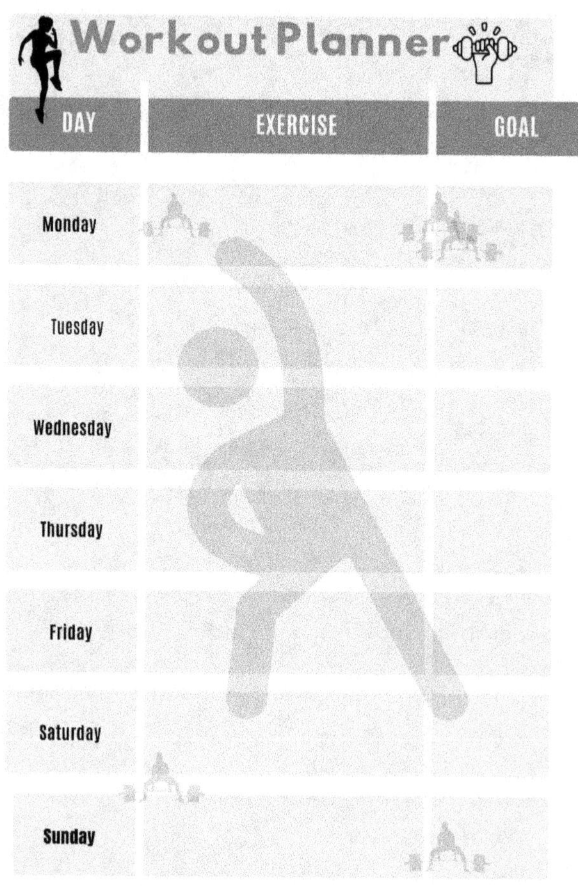

Workout Planner
DAY
EXERCISE
GOAL
Monday
Tuesday
Wednesday
Thursday
Friday
Saturday
Sunday

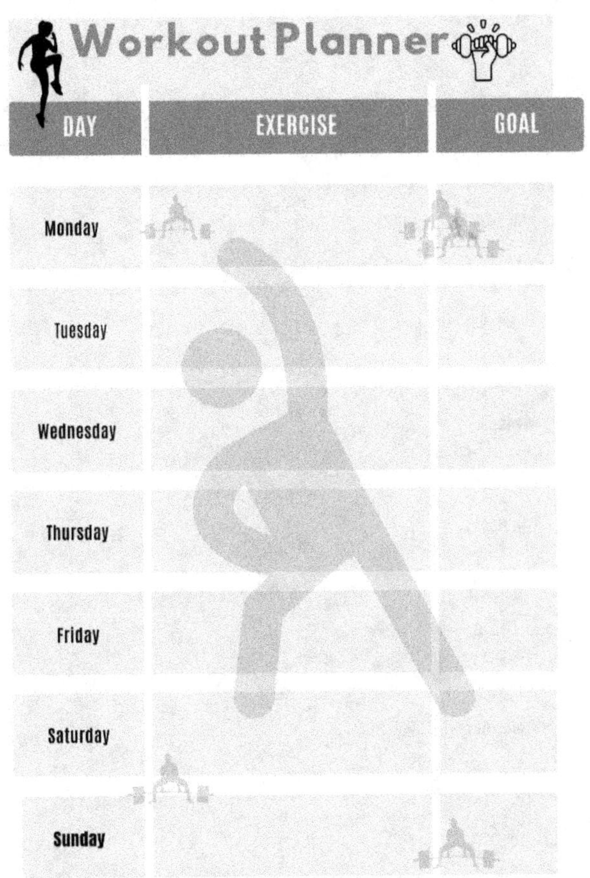

Workout Planner
DAY
EXERCISE
GOAL
Monday
Tuesday
Wednesday
Thursday
Friday
Saturday
Sunday

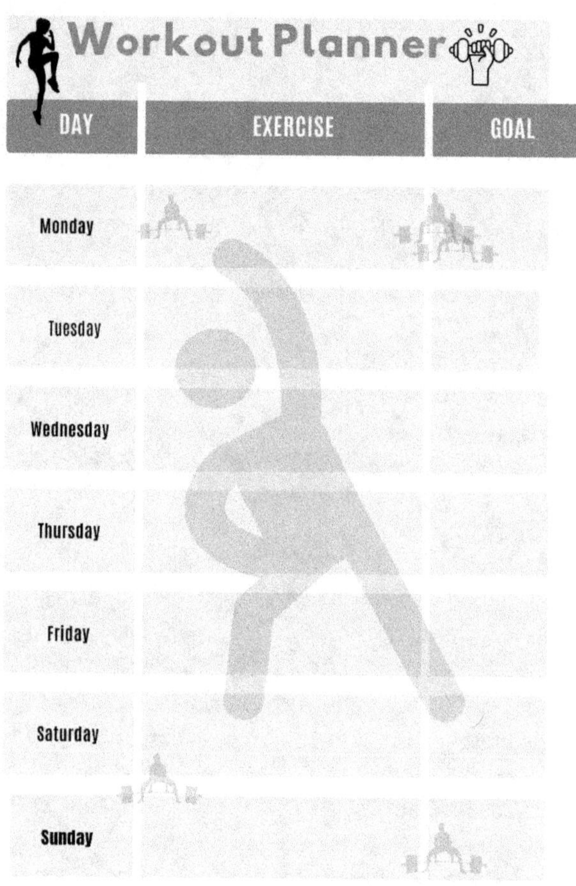
Workout Planner
DAY
EXERCISE
GOAL
Monday
Tuesday
Wednesday
Thursday
Friday
Saturday
Sunday

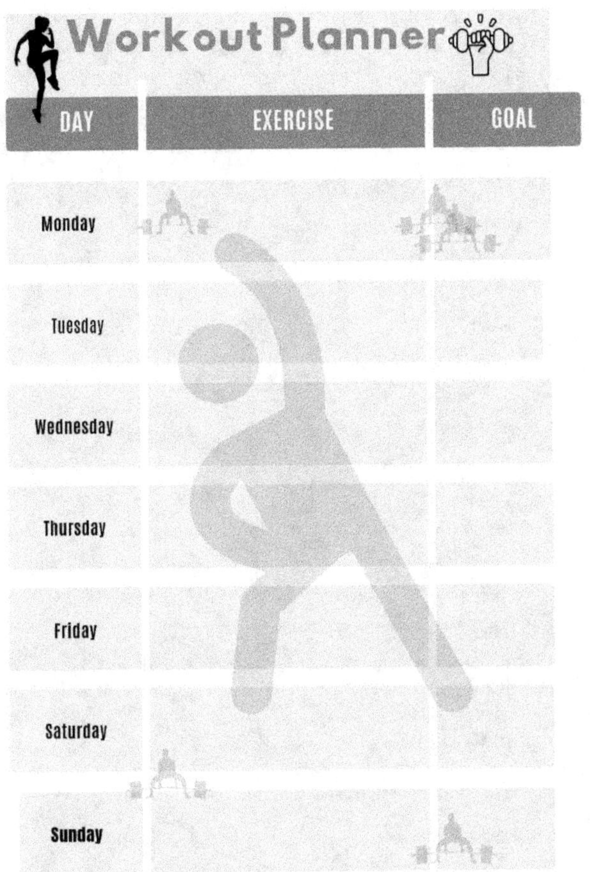
Workout Planner
DAY
EXERCISE
GOAL
Monday
Tuesday
Wednesday
Thursday
Friday
Saturday
Sunday

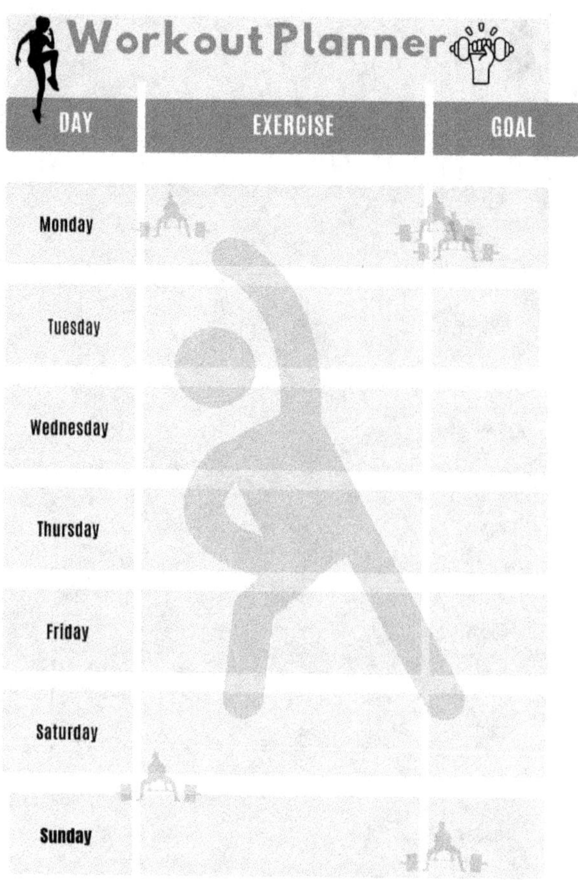

Workout Planner
DAY
EXERCISE
GOAL
Monday
Tuesday
Wednesday
Thursday
Friday
Saturday
Sunday

Workout Planner

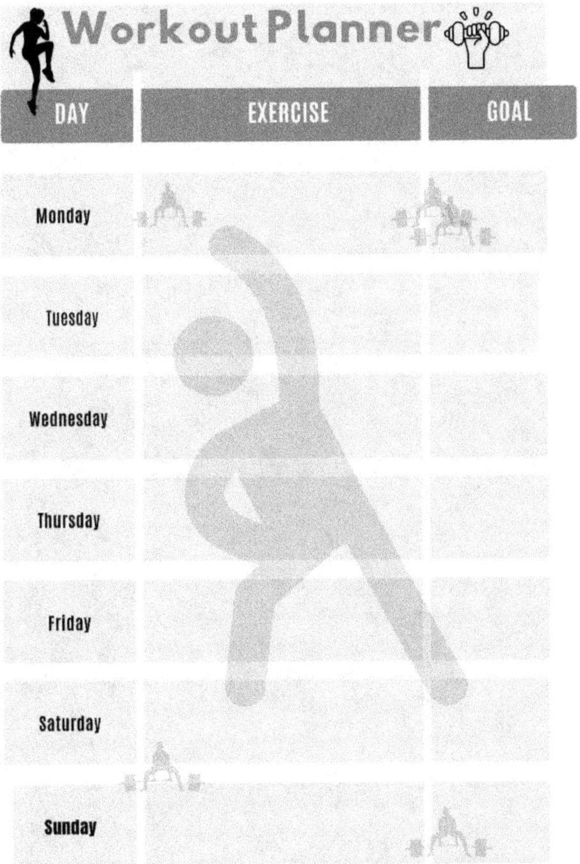

DAY	EXERCISE	GOAL
Monday		
Tuesday		
Wednesday		
Thursday		
Friday		
Saturday		
Sunday		

9 798878 365857